EMOTIONAL TRIAGE

A NURSE'S GUIDE TO

OVERCOMING BURNOUT
and
COMPASSION FATIGUE

OLIVIA LOVEJOY, RN

JOY RIDGE
P·R·E·S·S

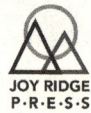

JOY RIDGE
P·R·E·S·S

Emotional Triage: A Nurse's Guide to Overcoming Burnout and Compassion Fatigue by Olivia Lovejoy

Copyright © 2022

Publishing and Design Services: MelindaMartin.me

Emotional Triage: A Nurse's Guide to Overcoming Burnout and Compassion Fatigue is under copyright protection. No part of this book may be used or reproduced in any manner whatsoever without written permission except in the case of brief quotations embodied in critical articles and reviews. Printed in the United States of America. All rights reserved.

ISBN: 979-8-9857080-0-4 (paperback), 979-8-9857080-1-1 (epub), 979-8-9857080-2-8 (audiobook)

Disclaimer: This book is not intended as a substitute for medical advice. The reader should consult a licensed medical professional in matters relating to his/her mental and physical health and particularly with respect to any symptoms that may require diagnosis or medical attention.

TRIAGE (NOUN)

The assignment of degrees of urgency to wounds (or illness) to decide the order of treatment amongst a large number that require attention

Origin—French (verb) Trier: To separate out

NEW OXFORD AMERICAN DICTIONARY

DEDICATION

TO MY COMRADES IN ARMS,
MY FELLOW HEALTHCARE PROFESSIONALS,

You are a continual source of strength and inspiration. You have been my teachers, my mentors, my friends. I am proud to be a member of your team. I am proud of the work we are doing. May we continue to persevere.

TO MY HUSBAND, JACOB,

You continue to demonstrate what love looks like in action. Thank you for enduring this crazy life with me. You are strong and steady, and you let me fly so high. Thank you, my love.

CONTENTS

1. First, Do No Harm To Yourself 1
2. How in the Hell Did I Get Here? 9
3. Keep Swimming Or You Will Drown 21
4. Energy 37
5. Emotional Stew 45
6. What is Compassion Fatigue? 49
7. What Self-Care Is, and What It's Not 55
8. Micro-Habits 63
9. Affirmations 67
10. Visualizations 79
11. Rituals 89
12. Quiet Headspace Time 93
13. Uncluttered Spaces 97
14. Avoiding Black Holes 101
15. Prioritize Sleep 105
16. Be Silly 107
17. Hydration 111
18. Personal Anthem 115
19. Dance It Out, Sing It Out 119
20. Get a Life 123
21. Renewing Your Purpose....................................... 133
22. So, Now You Know 135

Resources 141

Conclusion.. 149

CHAPTER 1

First, Do No Harm to Yourself

I see you. I see the weariness behind your eyes and the permanent furrow that has developed on your brow. I've followed your footsteps down long hallways to your patient's bedside. You are exhausted. But your patient is ever-present in your mind, and they need you. They need more from you. The responsibilities and expectations upon you just keep on coming. I know you keep a strong face on.

You were trained, like me, to push through. There are lives on the line here, after all. You do daily what the average person can barely comprehend, and you are called into action again. "Patient care comes first!" You use that motto as a pledge of honor. Often patient care comes before you pee, before you eat, and before you rest.

You work your shift, and you go home. But it doesn't feel like you ever left. Your shifts all run together. The work follows you home, and it won't allow you to rest. As you sleep, your subconscious is still rolling through your day. What did you forget to do? What detail did you fail to emphasize in your handoff report? It can be so hard to let go. What if you didn't do enough? You should have done more. What did you miss? What did you forget? What situations were so bad that they won't let you forget them?

There is a constant bombardment from your mind because what you missed is waiting for you in the darkness as you close your eyes tight and try to rest. It worms its way through your pillow and into your ear, and it whispers, "You're not good enough . . ." As if you needed a reminder. You may even have visions of patients you could not save and the people you have disappointed. You did your best. But your best wasn't enough. Sometimes it seems that your best may never be enough.

Let me ask you a question: What have you done to care for yourself today?

One of the first rules of healthcare is to "first, do no harm." We dutifully assume that this means doing no harm to the patients in our care. But this concept should not be exclusive to our patients. What if it also means first doing no harm to ourselves? We cannot help others if our health and energy are depleted. Let that sink in for a minute.

First, Do No Harm to Yourself

What is your health like? Be honest with yourself now. What is your mental health like? Really? What would you tell a patient like yourself? Are you getting enough sleep each night? Are you getting enough exercise? How are your relationships? How about your sex life, your personal time, your weight, or even your financial health? All these things and more make up your quality of life.

Have I lost you? The truth is, friend, most of us are lost when it comes to how we address caring for ourselves. We are very well trained in caring for others, and let's be proud of ourselves for that. But what I've witnessed over the last few years, especially through this pandemic, is that our self-care practices could use a bit of work. It can be a feat to juggle all the demands put upon us and still maintain a healthy state of mind and an open heart.

While I have been blessed with what I've been told is a blindingly optimistic disposition, just a few years into my nursing career, I was becoming one of those grumpy-ass nurses! You know the ones I'm talking about. As a new-ish nurse, I was struggling to adjust to the pressures of a career in healthcare while being a busy wife and mom. I noticed that I was succumbing to the negative energy and the negative people that surrounded me. I tried, but I couldn't shake the funk I was in. It got so bad that I didn't feel comfortable in my own skin. I was anxious and irritable. The sarcastic words coming out of my mouth didn't sound like me. "Ugh, this shit again today?" Even my self-talk (the voice I couldn't escape from) was whining. My outlook turned pessimistic. I didn't like who I was becoming. Worst of all, I felt my inner light going out. What had this career done to me in just a few short years? I wasn't enjoying my work. I felt like just another cog in the giant healthcare machine, detached from my purpose and bored with the endless tasks at hand.

I began to notice the same things in my coworkers. Some of them just seemed bound and determined to have a miserable day. They showed up for work already looking defeated. Was that what I had to look forward to? I couldn't help thinking, "Have I worked so hard for this new career and put in all this struggle and effort only to be this unhappy? To give and give, to empty myself, and to have nothing left for myself and my family?"

This was not the life I wanted. But I decided I was not about to give up on making nursing work for me. As a result, I read a lot. I cried a lot. I prayed and I searched for answers. I stood back and took a good hard look at my own life and my own (sometimes destructive) patterns and processes. I asked, "Why?"

What lies hereinafter are some of the answers and solutions I found for myself.

I love being a nurse. I am confident that I was called to be a nurse. But being a caregiver, in all its varieties, is really hard. We all throughout healthcare need to learn a better way to sustain ourselves and to support each other in doing so.

The purpose of this book is to challenge the conventional ways we think of caring for ourselves and to improve the way we manage our energy. Our energy is our greatest resource. I will help you rethink your self-care and to break it down into tiny, easy-to-do pieces, even when you're exhausted—especially when you're exhausted. These strategies I lay out for you in the following chapters are mostly just little tweaks and mind shifts to brighten your outlook and get your energy up off the floor. They are bite-sized methods to help you cope and to deal with some of the emotional baggage we all collect through the course of a day. Let's face it, pandemic or not, caring for the health of others is a tough life path. Most of the research done for this book I did to keep my own sanity, and I haven't completely lost my shit yet. So it must be working.

Emotional Triage

Disclaimer: I am not a psychologist, psychiatrist, counselor, or an individual trained in those specialized areas of mental health.

I am a woman, a nurse, a mom, a wife, and so many other things. I have a knack for putting all of myself into the things I am passionate about. I chronically overinvest myself. Also, I have a propensity for overthinking and not being able to disengage my mind or my heart. Sometimes this is to my detriment, as I am prone to burnout. I have burned out many times over the course of my forty-three years. But I am resilient, if nothing else. I am also a reasonably educated person of sound mind who has some ideas to share with you based on my hard-won experiences.

Also, let me state that I am nowhere near a self-care expert or a Zen-goddess type. The fact is, some days I really struggle to keep it together. I am a work in progress just like you. The job I do as a Registered Nurse is really hard. My personal life is as complicated and hectic as it is beautiful. But I am on a conscious journey to have more peace within me and to enjoy a healthier mental and emotional space. I work regularly on letting go of all the bullshit I encounter daily.

First, Do No Harm to Yourself

But it's hard, man! I have been known to utter "WTF" under my breath more times in a shift than I am proud of. Okay, maybe a few weren't under my breath. The only thing with a dirtier mouth than a sailor is a nurse on her fourth (or more) consecutive shift. Am I right?

If you know where I'm coming from, then this book was written for you, my friend! Welcome! You are exactly where you are supposed to be right now, reading this book. Settle yourself in and get comfortable. It won't be too scary, and it won't take too long. I'm glad you found me. I've got some good stuff to share with you here, so read on.

CHAPTER 2

How in the Hell Did I Get Here?

I work as an RN Clinical Supervisor of Surgery in my small community's trauma center. The nature of my job (and probably yours too if you're in healthcare) demands that I push back against circumstances that largely I cannot change. This job requires me to be a taskmaster, a ringleader, a problem solver, and an aspiring mind reader. (My crystal ball still hasn't arrived from Amazon, so I wait impatiently for it.) It is my job to make sure surgeons and anesthesiologists and surgical staff have the time, space, and resources they need to do their surgical cases, and when they don't, I fix it. Or I mitigate the damages and consequences. As you may imagine, all of this is easier said than done.

I manage the assignments and schedules of numerous nurses, scrub techs, and ancillary staff. I coordinate surgical care for trauma patients who need to go to the Operating Room urgently. If someone has a subdural hematoma, or an inflamed gallbladder, or any other ailment requiring urgent surgical intervention, I get the call to squeeze them onto the day's already busy schedule. I attempt to keep it all running on time with our regularly scheduled caseload. I try to keep everybody safe, sane, and happy. But the whole thing can turn into a dumpster fire so quickly. Often, no matter what I do, no matter how far I turn myself inside out, things don't go as planned. I still feel like I have failed. My efforts are too often futile.

The assortment of big personalities, patient acuities, and the speed at which the whole situation changes can be debilitatingly stressful. But, hey, I love this job! I'm basically the nursing equivalent of an air traffic controller. I get to affect many lives every day by doing what I do. When I do my job well, my surgical teams shine (I work with an amazing staff), physicians look good at what they do (many of them are really good anyway), and patients have more successful outcomes (isn't this the point?).

My desk in the middle of our surgical hallway has been referred to candidly as the "fire hydrant." It's where everyone comes to piss, whine, bitch, and to make their "recommendations." It is the ever-convenient location to off-load their complaints, problems, and issues. Just swing by and lift your leg. I will pay close attention and gladly take notes of your valuable input. Thank you! From an energetic perspective, this fire hydrant analogy isn't too far off. By the end of a tough day, I often feel like I've been pissed on—figuratively, anyway.

I didn't grow up dreaming of being a nurse. I sort of fell backwards into a nursing career. I remember my high school guidance counselor telling me I would be well suited for a career in nursing. I looked at her, betrayed, like she must not have understood me at all. I excelled at my science courses. I loved the experiments, especially the dissections. The physical body and its functions fascinated me. But back then, I knew I wanted to be a veterinarian. Animals were more emotionally safe. Being so innocent and trusting, they needed saving. I don't think I felt strong enough or capable—or worthy enough even—to work on people. Honestly, it never even crossed my mind. People were too emotional, too vulnerable, too real.

Looking back now, I see that I just wasn't ready. I had to get scuffed up a bit by life before I felt strong enough to take on caring for humans. It takes strength to look into the eyes of someone who is ill, injured, or experiencing a traumatic event. There is just too much raw truth there if you're not ready for it. Honestly, I think I was too scared to even consider the option, and I intentionally avoided human healthcare.

After six years, two junior colleges and two universities, I graduated with a bachelor's degree in Animal Science. Ok, so I took the long way around, and it wouldn't be the first time. Before I even graduated college, I knew I didn't want to be a vet. It didn't feel right anymore. I couldn't find my niche or decide on a specialty to pursue. I kept searching in vain for it. But the time had come where I had to pay the bills. All my years of education didn't really qualify me to do anything. Except to sell pharmaceuticals, or to marry a dairyman and help him take care of the herd in the milking barn. I didn't exactly do that, but I wasn't too far off. I married a rodeo cowboy, I took care of our horses (I was an avid rider), and I got my real estate license. It was right out of a country song. Real estate wasn't ever in my set of life goals, but I was good at it, and the money at the time was great.

Years pass quickly when you are young, fabulous, and caught up in an ever-escalating whirlwind of trying to prove yourself. Although I found myself on an unexpected path, the ten years or so that I practiced real estate were full of valuable learning experiences. Those years made me strong, even brave. I had to learn how to have tough, real conversations with clients about uncomfortable topics like money, debt, and estate planning. I learned to manage a client's expectations and helped them establish realistic expectations. I got yelled at, turned down, and got my feelings hurt. I sometimes made people unhappy with my words and my actions. I disappointed them when sales did not happen, and I did not crumble. I was growing stronger from the struggle.

Through those years I learned I really liked teaching and empowering people. I won when my clients won, and I got excited about that. I could see the impact that my insight and energy could have on a situation and on the lives of the people around me. I got into management and coached other real estate agents on making their sales. I was learning to be an advocate for others. But I hadn't figured out yet how to control or sustain my own energy or to advocate for myself, so these years were some of my first experiences with burnout and resilience. Also, I was starting to learn about setting emotional boundaries for myself. Mostly I learned this lesson by allowing those boundaries to get crossed, time and time again. But I think that lesson is finally sinking in.

Emotional Triage

It was a decade of extreme professional and personal highs and lows, much like the real estate market of that same time. It started with me growing up way too fast and taking on more personal and professional responsibility than any twenty-two-year-old is prepared for. I went from single college student to married successful realtor, with over $14 million in annual sales in just a couple of years. I literally wrote my final college paper from my private real estate office. In addition, the cowboy and I were partners in multiple development corporations, new parents to a baby girl, and building a big fancy home of our own. What could possibly go wrong?

What goes up must come down, as they say. The real estate roller coaster ride ended about ten years after it began, and so did my life as I knew it. I found myself with a failed investment company, a failed marriage to the cowboy, and a horse trailer filled with the expensive, useless crap I had accumulated over the course of our marriage. The horse trailer was parked in front of my studio apartment, where my daughter and I moved when I left the ranch. I still remember seeing my fancy business suits on the dirty floor of the horse trailer, dried horse shit scattered across the leg of my favorite silk pants. The image reeked of symbolism for how I felt about myself.

How in the Hell Did I Get Here?

I started from the beginning again. I was broke and aimless. I didn't know what I wanted to do; I just knew I couldn't do what I had been doing. The Great Recession, as we would call those years, had worn me out on sales of any kind. Most of my clients were builders or real estate developers who were broke, or going broke, or people who were upside down in their homes. The banks weren't negotiating with homeowners yet, still thinking they were too big to fail. It was heartbreaking. Real estate sales as I knew it was no longer an option for me. I just didn't have the heart for it anymore. My soul was tired. I was emotionally exhausted from all the strife. I felt defeated and even ashamed. Ashamed that I couldn't fix the problem my clients were in. But the real problem, the economy, was so much bigger than me.

I kicked around for a year or so trying to figure myself out and licking my wounds. I knew I had to keep moving forward. I had a daughter to set an example for. Those tough experiences, as a bonus, had left me with a slightly thickened skin, and a head and heart full of life lessons and skills. It was time to rally again. I felt it coming, like jungle drums beating inside me. I remembered my guidance counselor and how she urged, "You might make a great nurse." Something clicked and transitioned within me. I was inspired again to remake myself and to build my future.

I had missed the science, the research, and continuous learning. Also, those years of real estate had left me feeling empty, like I had whored myself out for a few bucks. A little extreme, I know. But I just felt like I was put on the earth to do something more meaningful. I wanted to make a difference to somebody, and in so doing, make a difference to myself. So back to school I went. Thankfully, I was only a half-hour commute from a top-ranked nursing and healthcare program at my local junior college (Go Cougars!). I didn't have to uproot my life, or my daughter's life, any more than I already had. I diligently started on my prerequisite coursework, and before I knew it, I had been accepted into the registered nursing (RN) program.

Life moved faster and faster after that. I met my now-husband who, in addition to being an amazing human, is a renowned local chef. We had two more girls, one born the year before nursing school, and one born during my last semester of nursing school. Whoopsie! I don't recommend going through nursing school that way, but I know that it can be done, and it can be done well. One of my proudest moments was graduating with honors in 2017 just two months after delivering my youngest daughter. I don't know that I had ever, up to that point, maintained that kind of focus. I just had to finish what I had started. It felt good to prove to myself that I could do it, especially with a couple little additions in tow. I was grateful, too, for the awesome people who supported me and my husband with childcare, dinner invites, and thoughtful words. Without their help, we would've struggled more getting through those short but challenging years. Never underestimate the power of your people.

The summer after graduation, I was lucky enough to get hired directly into the surgical department as a Circulating Nurse in the operating room. I loved it! I got to be someone's safe space in a scary time, a port in a storm. I immersed myself in it, working and learning as much as I could.

OR life is very specialized, a breed of nurse all its own. So it wasn't too long before I began feeling like I was pigeonholing myself too soon in my nursing career. I was losing some of my "nursey" qualities. You know, the basics like full body assessments, IV starts, medication administration, and heart, lung, and bowel sounds. These things are not generally part of the OR nurse's workflow. I started feeling like I wouldn't ever be able to assimilate with the regular nurse population if I didn't stop, start over (jeez, is this a theme?), and go back into basic nursing care. I loved the operating room, but I figured that if I had a year or so at least of critical care experience under my belt, then I could really go anywhere in my nursing career. So I took a position in our busy telemetry unit. I cared for post-ops, admitted trauma patients, patients experiencing substance withdrawal, lots of neuro patients, and so many other things. I liked it. The experience at the bedside with those patients validated me and made me more confident in my abilities and my intuition. I had a wonderful mentor, and I made some great allies within the hospital. It was an opportunity I likely never would have had if I had stayed working in surgery. I was thinking about beginning to orient into the ICU, where the real badass nurses work. I had even enrolled back in school to pursue becoming a Nurse Practitioner, but something else came up.

Out of the blue, a leadership position opened in the surgical department. One of my OR supervisors recommended I apply. She knew I had some management experience from my real estate days, had some experience working in other hospital departments, and that I hadn't burned too many bridges while making my exit from the OR. The first two times she asked me, I said, "No way." But she had planted the seed in my brain, and over the next several weeks

How in the Hell Did I Get Here?

I couldn't stop thinking of the opportunities of the position. I felt like I was uniquely suited for the job. So I went ahead and applied. They made me an offer, and I accepted the position.

CHAPTER 3

Keep Swimming Or You Will Drown

Barely six months into my new position as Clinical Supervisor in Surgery, we found ourselves on the verge of a global health pandemic. All elective surgical cases had been cancelled. Our daily surgical schedule, usually robust, had dwindled to a mere few cases a day. We were only doing cases where the urgency of the patient's need for surgical intervention overrode the risks for potential exposure. Intubation for anesthesia is an aerosolizing procedure, and we were dealing with an airborne virus, so the few surgeries we were doing became a high risk for my staff. The additional Personal Protective Equipment (PPE) needed to keep the surgical teams safe takes time to don and doff and makes it cumbersome to perform their duties within the sterile field. The protective barriers added an additional layer of difficulty to precarious surgical situations where tensions were already running high.

Emotional Triage

We lived days at a time in gloves, face shields, and N-95 masks—something I've become accustomed to. We were prepared at my little California hospital, almost hyper vigilant. We were waiting for the surge of the virus to afflict our community. We waited anxiously, almost impatiently. We kept hearing it was coming. We saw it making its way across the world. Devastation everywhere. First China, then Italy, New York, New Orleans, Phoenix. But not here yet?

When we left the hospital and went home, the pandemic was still largely misunderstood by our families and friends. "Is it real?" friends would ask me. "Is it really killing people here?" "It sounds like fake news. It is just the media just trying to scare us." The dichotomy between my personal life and hospital life was becoming wider and wider, as many people argued about mask mandates, their personal rights, and schools closing to stop the spread of the virus.

I felt anxious and conflicted inside. It was difficult to balance my understanding of the science and what I saw inside the hospital setting and the politics and posturing outside. Worse yet, I was idle and had plenty of time to overthink and over-feel the storm brewing around me. I watched the news and Facebook, videos about how nurses in Detroit and other cities were struggling. They were tremendously short-staffed with no one to relieve them from their shifts, and they were overrun with sick patients. And here I sat at home—not working—on the other side of the country. Another shift had been cancelled because there were no elective surgeries to do. I had just worked for a year cross-training in our Telemetry Unit. I had learned a lot that year. I was trained! Maybe I could do something to help? Sure, it wasn't ICU experience, but I could do something. I felt guilty doing nothing, just watching the drama unfold across the country.

I felt this uncomfortable knowing inside that I needed to be there, wherever "there" was. New York, Detroit, Phoenix, and other cities were becoming crippled in this health crisis and were begging for Registered Nurses to help them. Here I was, a happily married mother of three girls with a shiny new promotion to Clinical Supervisor. Nobody was expecting me to go anywhere. It wasn't even in my job description. But there it was, that nagging little feeling pushing me right into the deep end. It wouldn't go away. I couldn't stand waiting around anymore. I began realizing that I wanted to go fight this thing. Nurses are people of action, and the inaction was killing me inside.

I casually mentioned to my husband one morning about all the travel assignments I had seen posted in the COVID hot spots. I said in passing, "If I were single or didn't have kids, I'd be on a plane in a hot minute." I explained that I felt called to be there, to do my part, to do something. He said, "Well, what the hell is stopping you? I've got things handled here. Go! Go do your thing, baby." I felt both stunned and empowered by his statement. I made a couple of calls inquiring about how I could help, and the next thing I knew, I had an assignment and a plane ticket. It was literally that fast. I was taxiing down the runway and cleared for take-off just a few days later.

I spent twenty-four days in Detroit. I arrived mid-April 2020, about a month after the US had officially declared a pandemic. I arrived just after the big surge in Detroit. The place was surreal, like a scene out of some sci-fi movie or *The Walking Dead*. The streets of the grand city were mostly empty. The only other people in my massive hotel along the river were other nurses who had traveled from far and wide to help and some National Guardsmen who had been deployed to assist in the viral disaster. Their military vehicles convoyed from the hotel to their battle station a little farther down river.

We would leave the hotel in small groups to carpool to the hospital for our shifts, our own little calvary reporting for duty. Most of us wore our N-95s door to door. I put it on before I left my hotel room and didn't take it off until I passed over the threshold of that room again, some fourteen hours later. I didn't dare step into the hospital without my mask already on. Everything felt contaminated and probably was. Public surfaces could not be trusted. Doorknobs and countertops might as well have been lava. Touch it, and die. A little on the dramatic side, but a casual eye rub and I could have become infected. Pathogens are sneaky like that. And this one was proving to me every day that it could do some serious damage.

I was assigned to various departments within the hospital. Every day was a different department, on a different floor, and a different adventure. One day was the COVID-positive Medical Surgical unit, for those patients who had graduated ICU but were still really sick. The next day it was a "clean" (un-COVID) department. "Clean" was a misnomer, as we would discover several days into their hospital stay that some patients had never been tested in the first place. Nothing like finding out the patient you've been treating for the last two days is now in the COVID unit on a ventilator. It was easier mentally to just assume that everyone had it and get on with it. The logistics of the testing, the isolation protocols, and the Personal Protective Equipment were overwhelming the system and the staff. Mistakes were bound to happen.

I saw my share of COVID and the mess it was making inside the bodies of my patients. But I also saw patients afflicted with many other things. The acuity of the non-COVID patients often rivaled those in the COVID units. It is important to note that patients with diseases and ailments having nothing to do with COVID-19 were still needing care. With the world so focused on the pandemic, the fact that these "regular" patients were still coming through the emergency room and being admitted to the hospital is easy to forget. For nurses and other caregivers, the regular workload didn't go away; COVID just layered on top of what was already a busy and strained team of hospital staff. The amount and intensity of the work was tremendous. Most shifts felt like I was swimming upstream against a strong current. I was barely keeping my head above water.

I treated several patients who were post-op from a gunshot injury, of all things. I found this so sad; amidst the pandemic, this type of violence still rages on. I saw the most horrific of pressure ulcers in bed-bound patients who were transferred from long-term care facilities on lockdown. Other patients were suffering from chronic and untreated advanced renal disease. (Interestingly, I also started seeing patients who had recovered from COVID and had a new onset of renal disease.). Others were living with complications of AIDS, post-op amputations, advanced dementia, and a continuous undercurrent of ailments that are all too common to those of us involved in basic nursing care.

We tend to talk about these patients as diagnoses, as if dehumanizing them keeps them at arms-length from our emotions. It's a long-established coping mechanism, I think. But they are people. And man, they were scared to be in the hospital at that time. Most of my patients, the oriented ones anyway, felt certain they were going to catch COVID at the hospital. Some probably did. They were skeptical and untrusting of the medical system and the care I was giving them. This phenomenon was new to me. I found myself trying to educate and convince people that, medically, they needed to be in the hospital. There was so much fear. Honestly, I was scared too.

After a long day, I'd open the door to my hotel room and stand in a small corner of the entryway, so as not to contaminate my safe zone. I carefully kicked my shoes into a plastic bag. I would strip down and throw my dirty scrubs in a designated pile under the bathroom sink. I was mindful not to touch anything, as I had just handled all the clothes I had been wearing all day, and my hands were now potentially covered with the virus as well as a plethora of other pathogens. I could have infected myself. I stepped into the hottest shower I could tolerate, and I scrubbed. I ran the water in my eyes, mimicking an eye wash station. I blew snot rockets, just to dislodge anything I might have inhaled. I began to feel a bit obsessive. I emerged from the shower red and raw. I remained vigilant and guarded, even in the perceived safety of my hotel room.

I was grateful many times for my surgical training. It made my movements careful and intentional. My internalized basic sterile technique made my precautions more innate and instinctual. I could trust that my training and technique would keep me safe. And it did. I escaped Detroit without contracting the virus. I was tested several days after I returned home and was finally able to safely rejoin my family, after quarantining for several days, without fear of infecting them.

The things that I saw during my days in Detroit confirm the images you probably saw on the evening news the spring of 2020. It was like practicing medicine in a war zone. Or at least what I imagine medical triage might look like in a war zone. I have never served in the Armed Forces, but particularly after this experience, I have a deep respect for those who have served. It was utter chaos—too few resources, supplies, and people. Too many patients and complicated patients at that. The healthcare workers I saw worked under miserable, emotional angst. Their families, friends, and coworkers were losing their fight with COVID, right there in that hospital where they worked! But there they were, reporting for another shift. They showed incredible resilience like I had never seen, but it was taking a toll. They were exhausted, weary. They had little energy for niceties. Who could blame them? They largely ignored our little cavalry that came into work every day. They carried a very heavy load with no end in sight.

I was very aware working beside those nurses and aides that I got to leave that shit show. Soon I would be going home to the warm California spring and leaving the cold, windy, empty hellhole behind me. They would stay and soldier on because it was their home. It was their daily reality. I developed guilt around this. It was only by the grace of God that my little pocket of the world was not overrun with this virus—not yet anyway. I expect that I would stay and fight for my home, just as they have done for theirs.

Emotional Triage

I traveled to Detroit with an ICU nurse from my home hospital. She would share her heartbreaking experiences when we would pass each other in the hotel lobby now and then. What a badass she is, by the way, she and every other ICU nurse. She was handling three, sometimes four, ventilated patients at a time. She explained that they were having a hard time weaning patients off the vents once they were on them. These patients became perpetually sedated, suspended in time. Waiting to heal or succumb. The nurses celebrated every time they got someone off the ventilator. But the celebrations didn't come often enough. The nursing supervisor in ICU asked her to work nearly every consecutive day she was in Detroit, because there was such a great need for her and her skills. She could have stayed for six months and probably not done enough. She came home after her contracted time, like I did. Now we pass in the hall of our home hospital. There is a silent knowing between us, like a bond created on the battlefield. This must be something like what soldiers experience returning home while the war rages on—feeling guilty for leaving home and guilty for getting to come home.

Now that I am back home, in my surgical department, I am not intimately involved in bedside patient care. I'm one step removed. The drama I encounter daily is more related to interdepartmental friction and meeting the expectations and preferences of our surgeons. Largely this is stress that I have created within me to meet what feels like unmeetable expectations. But it is stressful just the same, and I have to struggle through it. I've noticed, though, that this stress doesn't have as much of a grip on me as it did before my experience in Detroit. It has begun to feel a little trivial in comparison. A wider perspective will do that, I suppose.

There was a simplicity of purpose about working amidst devastation like that. Despite the difficulty, it felt good to be a part of the effort. It was very clear what we were fighting against and why. We made do with the meager supplies that we had. There weren't any other options. I remember one shift, I had to open sterile drain sponges to clean up a patient after a bowel movement. (I laugh at myself now because I remember that I still opened them using sterile technique. The force of a well-ingrained habit!) There were no wipes and no linens. It was either the drain sponges or the one-ply toilet paper out of the employee bathroom. Hospital workers were getting creative with PPE too. I remember some using surgical bonnets as shoe covers. These are usually used to cover the hair on a patient's head as they go into the operating room. Or they would use the red and yellow no-slip patient socks over the top of their work shoes. Anything to not take the virus home on their shoes. My favorite, though, was when I was given the surgical orthopedic hood to wear as eye protection because they were out of face shields and goggles. It seemed ridiculous, but that was what was left. Caregivers took and used whatever they could to protect themselves. Hospitals provided whatever they could get their hands on, as creative and unconventional as it may have been, to keep staff safe. We were all doing the best we could at the time.

So many of our hospital supplies have been affected directly or indirectly by the virus, whether they are a heavily used supply like any kind of PPE (so we get what we get) or they are manufactured in a place where the workforce has been heavily infected. Either way, the supply chain has been greatly affected. Many things remain on back order. Even now, it is difficult to get all the supplies we need for our regular surgical schedule. When I'm met with people's disgust at the lack of supplies, or that their favorite surgical mask is out of stock, all I can do is shrug and say, "Cuz COVID." It is difficult to not be frustrated with them. I remind myself that they have no frame of reference. They didn't see what

Keep Swimming Or You Will Drown

I did. Every time I open a pack of drain sponges or 4x4s, I remember all the other more creative uses I came up with for them.

I came across a social media post shared by a nurse friend several months after I had returned home, and I was taken right back to that Detroit hospital in my mind. My life has moved forward, slowly, and I'm putting the experience behind me. But this post reminded me that others are still in the throes of it. Even now, with new variants emerging and staffing in crisis, it is more poignant than ever:

> We are still here. We are fighting. We are working harder than we ever have. We are exhausted, we are frustrated. We are frightened because we may take this (COVID) home to our loved ones. We are so emotionally and physically drained. We skip breaks and eat whatever is handy, just to keep us going. We come in early and go home late. We are doing the best that we can.
>
> —Author Unknown

Emotional Triage

When I read these words, I cried. I saw myself in them. I saw them in the eyes of my friends and comrades across the healthcare spectrum. We are a weary bunch. A ragtag crew, struggling to do the best we can. Some emotional triage is needed, to say the least.

Healthcare has always been a difficult career path. But now the stakes are even higher for us. We fight an uphill battle every day to ward off the emotional and energetic baggage of the life of service we have chosen. We end up burned out and empty. Where do we go from here? How do we carry on? Who is coming to relieve us?

This book is not about COVID. I believe there will be plenty written about it, and I don't wish to give it any more power than it has already taken from us. But COVID was part of my emotional and professional journey leading up to writing these words. It helped to forge me, to make me strong and unafraid. I believe many of my peers have also grown strong during this time. But we are tired and exhausted to our cores. I fear our resilience is slipping.

This is a unique opportunity for healthcare, and the rest of the world, to acknowledge that we need some healing. PTSD and other mental health issues are not unique to soldiers and law enforcement. I believe mental and emotional health crises are becoming ever more real to us too. Healthcare workers are not immune to these struggles just because we know how to heal others. Our training has been outwardly focused. It is time we focus inward. Patient care comes first, right? But who is healing us? It is time that we do the deep inner work of honoring ourselves, practicing authentic self-care, and healing our own emotional wounds.

I did not set out to write. I have never thought of myself as an author. I have even surprised myself with my voice and passion for this book. In fact, I have hesitated to mention it, or to even call myself a writer in certain social and professional circles. Who the hell am I anyway? But this book has formed within me. And now, I am both honored and obligated to give birth to it and to share it with you.

In this book are my strategies for sanity in this chaotic and sometimes traumatic life of service that I have chosen.

You are holding in your hands my emotional and energetic first aid kit.

These practices have helped my mental and emotional health amid this pandemic, and I trust they will help me far beyond it. I encourage you to try these simple things, again and again, until they become a part of you. They will lift your spirits, as they have done mine. I bet with some practice, you will find your thoughts and your energy shifted into a higher, broader perspective.

These little suggestions are simple to fold into your daily routine. I know that they will lighten your heart and help to refocus your mind and your purpose. Once refocused, you can continue to do the great things you do. Your patients need you, and we, your comrades in healthcare, need you too.

Most importantly, you deserve to feel good about yourself, and the awesome and powerful force that you are.

CHAPTER 4

Energy

Before we get too far, I want to talk about energy, and what I mean when I use that word, especially since I have used it numerous times already. Even though it is only six letters long, *energy* is a big word. There is so much meaning and importance crammed between those letters. It should really be broken into multiple words to better define its meaning. But since we are here reading and writing within the constraints of the English language, that one word *energy* will have to do.

The way I see it, we have two different types of energy.

First, there is the energy that is in you, the one you supplement with coffee and energy drinks to jet-propel you through to the end of the day. It fuels your physical body. This is the energy you are likely most familiar with. When this energy is low, you instinctively know to rest, sleep, or eat. The physical parameters of your body can only stretch so far without this physical supplementation. After a good night's sleep and a healthy meal, this energy has generally been restored. Your physical energy tank is full and your body is ready to rock and roll again.

The other type of energy is different. I will distinguish it by using a capital E for Energy. It has been called many names, among them passion, enthusiasm, spirit, will, inspiration, intuition—to name a few. I think it is all these things and more. At its core, it is Energy. This second Energy makes up *who* you are. It can be shapeshifting and elusive, but it is within you just the same. It is the power behind you.

You may not think of yourself this way, but you are a power source. You create and emit your own powerful force that influences others around you and what you experience in each situation. It fuels your emotions, your inner thoughts, and your instinctive actions. This Energy force can't be regenerated by sleep, rest, or physical indulgence. Many have tried to refill this Energy with alcohol, drugs, or expensive things and experiences. Yet they remain empty. I believe with some mindfulness, purposeful self-care, and connection with other people's good Energy, we can consciously refill our own Energy. But believe me, this takes some practice.

Energy

These two types of energy constitute a kind of currency to us. We can choose where to spend them. Like money, they can be spent wisely, or they can be pissed away. Sometimes we are completely mindless about what we are spending our Energy on. Like those sneaky recurring charges that hit your bank account every month, Energy leaks can drain your tank without your even being aware of them. The trick is to be mindful of what you are choosing to spend your Energy on and to be on the lookout for situations where you are mindlessly spending it.

Examples of mindless Energetic spending include too much social media, gossip, or involving yourself in drama that has nothing to do with you. Additional ones are over-investing yourself in something (worthy or not), over-empathizing, and working too hard to please others. These sneaky Energy leaks can be very expensive to your overall well-being.

This is where it becomes so important to learn to check in with yourself. Think about and feel what your gauges might be reading on your respective energy tanks. Is your low fuel light on and you haven't even noticed? Only, instead of risking being stuck on the side of the road and out of gas like you would be in your real car, energetically speaking you have chosen to put your Energy pedal to the floor, hung

Emotional Triage

a left and are now speeding down Burnout Lane toward a fiery energetic crash. Likely your body is giving you signals, but you have been ignoring them. Listen to your body. Be open to acknowledging its signals.

I have noticed that my body warns me I'm running down Burnout Lane with sleeplessness, mental restlessness, fever blisters or sores in my mouth, irritability, and impatience with myself and my situation (and anyone unlucky enough to be around me.) Sometimes these things can be situationally explained away. I dismiss them or ignore them and suffer the consequences. Other times, all the signs are there and I am tuned in and paying attention to my energetic needs. I am able to downshift and coast into some rest and self-care. Burnout crisis averted. Until you become aware and mindful of the status and usage of your energy tanks (yes, both of them), you will continue to waste your precious Energy, time, and effort on things that are not worthy of your strife.

Even things that are worthy of your effort can cost a lot of Energy, and this is where it gets a little tricky. Should you work that extra shift? Your team really needs you, and they are short-staffed tonight. You want to help them out. But do you have enough Energy to give? Maybe you do. Are you in tune with yourself and listening to the signals your body is giving you? Has your low fuel light been on trying to get your attention? Or do you just need a good nap to set you straight again? Only you can know this. The more Energy you need to give, the more intentional you need to be about saving and replenishing your energetic reserve.

Good Energy can be cultivated, and here is how: use your purposeful intention to shift your thoughts, your emotions, and your actions. Once you figure this out (and believe me, this is an acquired skill), this will increase your Energy. I have good days and bad days with my Energy cultivation. But I've noticed that the more positive thoughts and Energy I cultivate, the more goodness and positivity I attract. I notice this difference in my surroundings, my coworkers, and in my own energetic perspective. It just feels better when you are surrounded by good Energy. You will become accustomed to the elevated feelings and emotions that positive Energy provides. Friends and coworkers may have an improved attitude from working close to you and the good Energy you provide.

A word on receiving another's Energy:

The affliction that can come from another's Energy is generally unintentional. Most people don't go around with the awareness of the idea of Energy sharing. But have you ever noticed how someone's bad mood can rub off on you? You've undoubtedly heard the popular phrase "misery loves company." Or how about this one, "birds of a feather flock together"? Do you notice how negative people often seem to hang out with other negative people? It's like they feed off each other, right? Well, they do. They keep sharing and affirming each other's negativity, and it grows stronger. Together, it's like their Energetic volume is turned up. Positive people seem to gravitate to other positive people too. They affirm each other's positivity and make their working environment more enjoyable for everyone.

Once you realize the power your Energy has in effecting change upon another person, you are responsible for using it appropriately. No more spewing a bad attitude all over the room. Some things just shouldn't be shared. My hope is to empower you to make your internal Energy more powerful than the external Energetic forces surrounding you. Hold your own rhythm and maintain your objectivity within the situation. This is not an easy thing to do. You will still struggle with your own reactions and needs. The first step is to just be aware of your own emotional responses and the resulting Energy generated within you. Once you are aware and acknowledging your emotional reaction, you can choose to respond differently.

Challenging things will still happen in your life, of course. But you will become less inclined to lose your power in those situations. You can become aware of the people and situations you are giving your Energy away to. Be selective with this!

We will talk more about how to cultivate your good Energy, ways to save it, and methods to protect your Energy in upcoming chapters.

CHAPTER 5

Emotional Stew

I think that many people who are attracted to a career in healthcare are sensitive to the Energies of others. They can naturally sense what others need, and they often want to fix it or lessen the burden. Healthcare is a calling, a spiritual mandate, even, for some. Most caregivers are naturally empathic. They take on the Energetic burdens of people in need as well as carrying their own. It can be a very heavy load. Patient after patient, shift after shift, we collect the traumas of those in our care and we carry them within us.

I learned early on in my nursing career that I had to learn to deal with these traumatic emotions and accumulated Energies. While I am very steady under the acute pressures of the moment, I tend to carry the Energy of the event away with me. It buries itself deep under my skin where it can hide. I carry it until I can find a safe space where I can carefully and intentionally unpack it from where it has been shoved deep down inside me. Then, when no one is looking,

Emotional Triage

I can cry if I need to. There, I said it. I cry. I am a crier. I've noticed that when I am carrying too heavy a load, my tears are much closer to the surface. They will even sneak up on me unexpectedly because I have not taken the time to deal with the Energetic burden I have been carrying.

Nearly every day, I encounter some new trauma and the corresponding Energy of each patient in need. Every time I roll a new mother emergently into the operating room, I fight back a few tears. She is hemorrhaging after her efforts to bring a new life into the world. Her blood is everywhere. I tell her, "You are safe, you are in good hands, we are here taking care of you." I can't say this without a lump forming in my throat. I stop short of saying, "You're gonna be ok, it will all be ok." I will do everything in my power to make sure that she is ok. But I know it is not a guarantee I can make. I have learned patients like her can go really fast. So I stop myself short of making promises I can't keep, and I feel the tears trying to push through. But the work is there, and it is always dependable. I diligently work her case. She is covered in drapes now. I forget her face, and the fear and exhaustion I saw in her eyes, and how she squeezed my hand for reassurance. I work faster, run for blood, and prime the line. Turn up the suction, open

Emotional Stew

more instruments. I appreciate the work. I can get lost in the tasks. The emotion has passed by now, overruled by the need for quick action.

Raw emotions like these are part of what make me a good nurse. They are part of what makes you good at what you do too. These traumatic emotions and memories can be painful for us and difficult to process. But they keep us human, and they bind us to the needs of our patients. That emotion and its corresponding Energy must go somewhere. It bubbles up within us whether we acknowledge it or not. Brewing and stewing deep down inside of us. Some of the ingredients of this emotional stew are fear, pride, frustration, pain, fatigue, doubt, powerlessness, and a million other unidentified, jagged emotions. Some emotions are fresh new experiences; others are nameless and rank from our neglect. We work in an industry of trauma, pain, illness, and suffering. People often meet us on the worst day of their lives. Some of the emotions we encounter throughout our workdays are inevitable for the situation. Big and powerful emotions are the uncomfortable but natural response to a traumatic event. They keep us poised for action. With training, they even keep us, and our patients, safe since we can anticipate what's next. We cannot change these emotions. But if we are not careful in dealing with them, these emotions day after day can begin to change us.

You may uncharacteristically begin to feel a lack of empathy or concern for your patients and coworkers. You may even feel resentful of your responsibility for their needs. You feel like you can't do it anymore. You are tired of pouring yourself out for them again and again. You are running on empty, and your give-a-shitter is sputtering out. These are a few common symptoms of compassion fatigue.

CHAPTER 6

What is Compassion Fatigue?

It has been said that compassion fatigue is the "cost of caring for others," and to me this feels about right. The phrase, as originally coined by Carla Joinson in 1992, defines the point when nurses lose their "ability to nurture." Then Charles Figley, a psychiatrist, redefined it in 1995 into a more clinical definition, linking it to a secondary traumatic stress disorder. Either way, if you have been working in healthcare in the last few years, you likely know what compassion fatigue feels like, even without any official definition.

Compassion fatigue was defined by Walker and Avant in their text *Strategies for Theory Construction in Nursing, 4th Edition* as "the physical, emotional and spiritual result of chronic self-sacrifice and or prolonged exposure to difficult situations that renders a person unable to love, nurture, care for or empathize with another's suffering." Compassion fatigue, and its bitchy little sister burnout, are robbing healthcare workers of their passion and Energy. But since you're the one reading this book, you probably already knew that.

If you have never heard of compassion fatigue before, I anticipate you will hear it quite often from now on. I had not heard about it either until I started researching. But I anticipate that compassion fatigue will reach buzzword status in the next couple years, as the emotional fallout of our healthcare staff begins to demand attention. This generalized awareness is good news for those of us in the trenches! As a diagnosis-driven group, we may finally have a name for our struggle.

Healthcare workers are just the tip of the spear, though. The term is recently being applied more broadly to teachers, shelter workers, and others who find themselves in continuous care or continuously caring for a cause. So we are in good company. Over one-third of Americans are a caregiver to someone such as a parent or a child. Of course, in healthcare, it is our job to care for others.

Patricia Smith of the Compassion Fatigue Awareness Project explains in her TED Talk a few other notable symptoms of

What is Compassion Fatigue?

compassion fatigue. Among them are emotional outbursts (anger, tears, frustration), physical ailments (chronic headache, backaches), desire for isolation, apathy and sadness, substance abuse, and self-medicating. Do any of these sound familiar to you?

Individuals with certain personality traits are also more prone to developing compassion fatigue. Those with an overdeveloped sense of responsibility, personal boundary issues, an impulse to rescue others, and individuals with unresolved pain and personal trauma have a higher risk for developing compassion fatigue. This list reads to me like a job description for healthcare, first responders, and the military too! What do we do when the heroes and warriors need help?

Seriously, what do we do about it? Are we hopelessly doomed? Is there a cure for compassion fatigue? Well, maybe. As you may have guessed, it's a little more complicated than taking a pill or having the pain and exhaustion excised from your chest and starting over unscarred. Like so many processes within our bodies and minds, our individual solutions are complex and varied. There is emotional and Energetic work required, and time is required to dig out of the hole created inside you from burnout or compassion fatigue. This is difficult to accept when you are already depleted and you would rather do anything else than show up for your next shift.

This is where I tell you that if you are in too deep, you should seek help, phone a friend, and a mental care professional. I have also listed some resources for mental health at the end of the book. If you still have your head above water, just barely, you may find some solutions in the pages that follow. But the cure? What about the cure for compassion fatigue?

Honestly, I believe the word *cure* is a misnomer in this case. According to Webster's, *to cure* is "to restore health, soundness, or normality." But this indicates going back to how you used to feel, like "normal." And what is that exactly? Our experiences change us and teach us. We become a different version of ourselves, with more perspective, after passing through the dark veil of burnout and compassion fatigue. I don't think we will ever return to normal after that experience. But we can heal and rebuild a more resilient and self-aware version of ourselves, one that can sniff out when we are nearing the edge of our resolve and help us to ease our way back from the tipping point. We can learn to

What is Compassion Fatigue?

adjust our grip on the hard things, take a breath, and then carry on with the understanding that "this, too, shall pass."

Really, it is the prevention of burnout and compassion fatigue that can be both cure and prophylaxis. It is taking conscious action and effort to care for yourself and to place appropriate boundaries around your Energy.

I know, you've been told about the importance of self-care before. Yeah, blah, blah, blah, self-care. But I promise, self-care is so much more than facials, naps, and running on a treadmill three times a week. There is a whole aspect of self-care you have probably missed, and it may be the secret to your healing.

CHAPTER 7

What Self-Care Is and What It Isn't

We've all heard a billion times the importance of practicing self-care. Well-meaning people say, "What you need is some self-care" all the time. Honestly, I hate this phrase. It's said as though self-care is the cure for whatever ails you. Is self-care so easy then? Should I already instinctively know what to do? Why does it feel so hard to get it right and to maintain it? Why do I keep screwing it up? What if it is our idea of self-care that is flawed and not self-care itself?

Let me summarize the basics of the self-care model we are all accustomed to: you've got to exercise 3–5 times per week, because we all know cardio is where it's at. Eat small healthy meals, several times a day. Not too many calories. That's the only way to sustain your energy and avoid burnout. Drink water, avoid alcohol (cough). Get pedicures and massages regularly. Do yoga, become really bendy, and learn to meditate. Reduce the number of stressors in your life (yeah, right; who can actually do this?). Take an expensive vacation. Reward yourself with a shopping spree. Indulge yourself—you work hard and you deserve it. "Because you're worth it, baby!"

If you're like me, all that sounds overwhelming, expensive even. With all the self-indulging, cardio-ing, meal planning, and yoga, where do I find the time and energy to do the normal things that life demands of me? Where do my kids and my bills and my dirty laundry fit into this self-care stuff? Or more appropriately, where does this self-care stuff fit in around them? I don't really have time for this idealistic version of self-care on a regular basis. Also, are those things really going to make me feel better long term? Are they sustainable in my real-world life? This idealistic version of self-care just feels like more unrealistic expectations on me as well as ramped-up consumerism, just another list of to-dos to self-loathe over and spend too much money on, something I can work on for a few weeks in January, then feel like crap about all year long. Inevitably, it's not self-care at all.

Let me nudge you into a different perspective on self-care. What most of us don't acknowledge is that there are multiple aspects of self-care. Self-care is as big and dynamic as you are. Just like there are multiple facets to your sparkling personality, there are multiple ways to care for your well-being. Of course there are! Self-care is not one size fits all or even one thing that fits you every day. Only you will know which type of self-care will be the most restorative to you on any given day, based on your own self-awareness and your needs for regeneration. Also, not all self-care feels good at the time. Sometimes it is delayed gratification. Accepting delayed gratification is top-shelf adulting!

Below, I have described these different aspects of self-care as levels. I find the idea of levels a reasonable way to organize this concept. It provides a mental visualization of a generalized hierarchy of ways to care for yourself. You can move up and down these levels very easily, and you should. But they are all equally important to sustaining you long-term. Allow me to introduce these to you.

Practical Self-Care

This includes exciting things like folding laundry, paying your bills, cleaning your house, and scheduling a doctor's appointment for yourself. These things are often not thought of as self-care. These little practical tasks, if left undone, can have a profound impact on the quality of your life. They nag at you. They feel like chores and errands. But they are the foundation of a stable and healthy life. With these basics done, life runs a little more smoothly.

Physical Self-Care

Honoring and maintaining your physical body. This of course includes, but is not limited to, regular exercise. Massages, pedis, haircuts, and even naps are all included in this category. This is most commonly what we think of as self-care. But without acknowledging and addressing the other levels of self-care, these physical methods will lack depth and won't be nearly as effective.

Social Self-Care

Enjoy connecting with others by nurturing your relationships. These connections can be light and transient or very deep, depending on the level of the relationship. Both can be so enjoyable. Sometimes sharing your Energy with others can feel really good. It can be so powerful to connect Energetically with another. Find others with good Energy and share Energy abundantly. You will both come away from the encounter with more Energy than you started with. Often, we build strong connections with people who are enduring the same struggle we find ourselves in. We can encourage each other.

Mental Self-Care

This category can be somewhat broad. Basically, it means anything that stimulates your mind and keeps you growing and curious. It could be learning something new, doing a challenging crossword, creating art, or even planning something. Your mind is a bit like a border collie puppy. It likes to work and to be challenged. Give it something to chew on so it doesn't get bored and, like the puppy, gnaw a leg off the coffee table (or some other equally destructive outlet).

Emotional Self-Care

This is a big one. It involves taking time to feel, acknowledge, and process your emotions, checking in with yourself, and honoring where you are today within that journey. Nurturing your emotional intelligence is here on this level too. And this is where you may begin to foster broader perspectives from what you thought you knew. Be open to the changes. Journaling can be a great way to unpack your emotions and to help you reflect and learn from your past as well as choose an authentic direction for your future.

Spiritual Self-Care

Spiritual self-care connects you to your higher power. This is not necessarily religious, although some people think of being spiritual as being religious. This level includes prayer, meditation, even communing with nature—whatever makes you feel connected, grounded, and fosters your self-awareness. Your intuition lives here on this level too. Be open and ready to receive a download when it comes along.

Notice that these levels are loosely correlated with Maslow's Pyramid. No, not the food pyramid—the one about the human hierarchy of needs. Please note that these levels of self-care are not listed in order of importance. Rather, they are loosely ranked by frequency of need. For example, you must sleep (physical) more often than you need to gather with friends (social). Also, in theory, you must eat (physical) more often than you pray (spiritual) or commune with your higher power, although I recommend prayer as often as possible.

What Self-Care Is and What It Isn't

Slide up and down these levels often and do something to care for yourself from each level. Approaching your self-care this way will make you feel rested, centered, and more regenerated. It is a genuine and holistic approach to caring for all of you. It is more manageable, more complete.

Many of the suggestions in this book can serve multiple levels of self-care. As you read on, think about what level each suggestion may provide for you. They can be totally individual. One person's social self-care may be another's mental self-care, depending on your intention and your emphasis. You decide. The point is that you show up and advocate for yourself by taking care of your needs on each self-care level.

It is very important also to acknowledge the intention behind your self-care as you perform each self-care action. It is almost like you are sending yourself a message: "See? You matter! You are worth taking care of and I am doing this for you." Affirm it to yourself: "I am taking action to honor myself." By doing this, each intentional act of self-care reinforces your worthiness, and you become consciously aware that you have done something kind for yourself. When things are done consciously, they are harder to forget.

Emotional Triage

As a side note, I totally acknowledge the benefits of regular exercise, healthy eating, and occasional self-indulgence. But I feel the way we have been taught to go about obtaining the benefits of these traditional self-care activities is unsustainable for those of us who are nearing burnout. It is too often task-driven and mindless. It adds to our burdens instead of helping us to release them. This sets us up for failure in the long term. Read on, and I'll explain more in the next chapter.

CHAPTER 8

Micro-habits

One of the predominant themes behind the remainder of this book is the micro-habit. If this is a new concept for you, I am so pleased to introduce it. The idea of the micro-habit is to make daily goals so small, so simple, that a reasonable person would find it unreasonable to talk themselves out of doing it. Small efforts over time yield big results. Often, mental barriers surrounding beginning keep us from starting. Micro-habits help to reduce this barrier. Since the immediate goal is so small, you almost trick your mind into overcoming the mental hurdle of starting. This concept was made popular by James Clear in his great book *Atomic Habits*, and it really has changed the way I approach my personal goals and day-to-day tasks and transformed the way I think of my self-care.

Almost every January, we start rolling out the resolutions and making some big goals. I love a big hairy goal and the prospect of making positive changes. I'm kind of a personal growth junkie. But I have the hardest time making those big changes stick. I start out so strong, but then I lose steam and revert to my old habits. Maybe you do this too? "I need to get in shape," you say to yourself, "so I must start working out." This can be daunting. You strategize a workout plan, maybe join a gym. You're really feeling motivated this time. You even bought yourself some new workout gear. Nothing says dedication like some new yoga pants.

Time goes by and you are enjoying your regular workouts. Then one day, not so far into your new plan, life happens. You don't work out. You just don't feel like it. You're tired. You're running late. You worked out really hard last time. Believe me, your mind will find any reason why you can't work out. It just sounds too hard today. All the excitement and motivation behind your new get-in-shape plan has waned. Motivation will do that; it dissipates over time. This leaves you feeling flat, fat, and defeated. Cue the downward spiral of self-shame. Damn it! You're right back where you started, looking up at another big, hairy, unattainable goal. Does this sound at all familiar to you? This is the story of my life.

Conversely, a micro-habit approach to working out is to commit to doing five squats every day. Ridiculous, I know,

Micro-habits

but five is all you have to do. You can do more, and maybe you usually will. But you will always do at least five. Easy, right? That is the point—it is easy. You don't even need to put on those new yoga pants or running shoes to do a few squats! Now you may be saying, "Nobody is going to get in shape by doing only five squats every day." Yeah, you may be right. But there is a strong chance that over time you will do more than five, and that you will do more than five consistently. The consistency, and the development of the habit, is the real goal. The key is to become someone who exercises regularly, and as a result you can achieve the benefit of being in shape. The habit must be established first, and a small habit can get you there.

Continuing with our example, there will be days when you don't want to do any squats. All the familiar excuses will come flooding into your mind. But, come on, it's only five squats. You only committed to doing five squats. The goal is so small that you really can't talk yourself out of doing it. Even if you do five squats in your pajamas as the last thing before you climb in bed, you did them.

Weeks, even months, go by. You're still doing your squats! You are meeting your small daily goal. You are keeping your

Emotional Triage

word to yourself and proving your self-worth. This behavior becomes self-honoring, and it builds upon itself. You are becoming someone who exercises regularly. No more shame spirals from non-performance. You begin to feel good about your follow-through. You are establishing a habit of behavior. When you take on a habit and it becomes part of your routine, you don't have to think too much about it. You just do it. When you don't have to think about it, it doesn't feel like you are even trying. Trying burns a lot of Energy, and sometimes physical energy too. We are in Energy-saving mode here.

Where in your life can you apply a micro-habit goal and couple it with a level of self-care? I bet there are a lot of places if you think about it. Everything from the five-squat method (physical self-care), to doing two minutes of dishes that have piled in the sink or three minutes of vacuuming Ritz crackers off the floor (practical self-care), or one minute of quiet reflection by yourself (spiritual or emotional self-care). You can find many, many uses for this handy tool. You might be surprised at the big impact of small and regular improvements in your life. Keep these micro-tricks in mind as we move on.

CHAPTER 9

Affirmations

"What you think about, you bring about."—Mom

The concept of affirmations is probably not a new one to you. Affirmations have been around forever and have been gaining popularity in the last couple decades. Before you discount them as just a way to blow sunshine up your own ass, hear me out.

My mom, a very wise woman, always told me, "What you think about, you bring about. Garbage in, garbage out." Now, I know that Mom was not the first, or only important person, to use this phrase. But she was the first important person to me. Even now, I can hear her sweet voice saying these words with determination and certainty. What Mom was saying was to be careful about my self-talk and about what "garbage" I allowed into my mind. She was warning me that my self-talk ultimately would influence my thoughts, my emotions, my habits, and my actions. So she empowered me to only put the good stuff in. And now I'm empowering you to do the same. Thanks, Mom!

It turns out that my mom is pretty smart. Science shows us that affirmations done regularly and repeatedly can change how your brain is wired together. Repeated thoughts and affirmations become like a well-traveled road that your mind can wander down when it is not sure where else to go. The ruts in the road become deep from repeated travel, and they carry you closer to the safety of your positive head space.

Our neurologist friends would refer to these roads as neural pathways that have been established between neurons after a repetitive action or thought. You may have heard the neurology concept that "neurons that fire together wire together." This concept is known as Hebb's Law, and it relates to how our brains bundle neurons that are commonly used together to automate and simplify our thought processes, thus reducing energy expenditure. Our minds reach for the familiar and repeated thought pattern because it is easier. Our brains are kind of lazy like that, and who can blame them? It is hard to think with focus all the time. But here's the kicker: you and I get to decide the thoughts that become easy and familiar. By regularly repeating your

Affirmations

affirmations, you are literally training your brain which thought to grab when it goes into autopilot mode. Make it something positive and useful that can better your situation.

I've noticed that without training my mind to reach for the more positive thought, it automatically goes to the dark side. I bet yours does too. The negativity is too easy, and it feeds on itself. It is your mind doing its job and protecting you from potential negative consequences. So be careful not to let that garbage infiltrate in. You are the keeper to the gates of your mind. Do your best to fill it daily with thoughts and affirmations to promote your well-being. Your mind believes everything you tell it. It hears everything you say. Protect it like you would protect a toddler's ears from your drunk brother's tirade of profanity. Earmuffs!

Seriously, though, there is some real neuroscience emerging on the power of the mind and its ability to change and adapt to the stimulus it is given. This is the concept of *neuroplasticity*, and it underpins the science around "what we think about, we bring about."

In her 2019 book *The Source*, neuroscientist and psychiatrist Tara Swart says, "Our brains are constantly evolving, refining, and learning in response to everything that we experience. We need to be aware of this and manage what we expose our brains to and how we deal with the impact. We can do this in real time, overwriting past hurts and cleaning up what is present."

Affirmations are a great way to engage neuroplasticity and train our brains to begin to overwrite the automated programs our minds have adopted in the past. I have written several affirmations for you. In all transparency, though, I wrote them for me. That is how this whole thing began. I started searching for affirmations that resonated with my situation. I wanted to give myself some positive thoughts and have them easily accessible when I felt the negativity caving in on me. I found some good ones, but some of them were just crap. I actually searched on Amazon for "affirmations for nurses." There were very few to choose from. The particular audio track I downloaded was ridiculous. One of the affirmations was seriously something like, "I follow the doctor's orders without question." I laughed myself right out of my meditative state. Clearly not written by a nurse!

Use these affirmations I have written to get you started. They don't take very long to do. Make a micro-habit out of them. Think about what level of self-care doing these affirmations help you honor. Are they spiritual self-care, or

Affirmations

more mental or emotional self-care? There is not a correct answer to this question. By asking this question, I am encouraging your mindfulness. For me, affirmations fall on my spiritual and emotional self-care levels. I do a few minutes of affirmations when I wake up, on my breaks at work, and sometimes just before I fall asleep. Some days, if I feel I need the extra mental support, I listen to my affirmation track on Audible on my commute to work. I also found a great app called Manifest. It pushes affirmations to my phone's home screen based on my preferences. I really enjoy it. Great affirmations pop up right in front of me when I least expect it. Also, try your hand at writing some affirmations that are specific to you and your situation. The more personal they are, the more they will resonate with your Energy. The more of your Energy you put into these, the more you will get out of them.

So how do you *do* an affirmation most effectively? Excellent question. Here's the best way I know.

As you read these affirmations, internalize them. Feel them as you read. Send your Energy into the nooks and crannies of the words. Say them out loud so you can hear them too! Repeat them individually. I usually say an affirmation twice before moving on to the next one. The repetition and the intention is key. Some affirmations may be more profound for you from day to day, so spend some extra time with these.

I've put these affirmations into two generalized categories: Pre-Shift/Mid-Shift and Post-Shift. They are designed to put you in the right mindset for each timeframe, but nothing here is rigid. So if you need an affirmation from one category or another, use it. Use it with abandon!

When you first get started, you may feel a little weird, like you are talking to yourself because, well, you are. Get over it and keep going. Nobody can hear you, right? It's just you and your mind in here. This is your sacred space and time.

AFFIRMATIONS

Pre-shift/Mid-shift

I am grateful for another day to make a difference.

∎

I am grateful for my place in healthcare.
It is a privilege to influence the lives
of my patients and their families.

∎

The work I do is important.
Not many people can do what I do.

∎

I may not be able to change the outcome for my patients,
but I can usher them through their journey
and keep them safe and comfortable.

∎

I am appreciated.

∎

Every day I am reminded of the blessings in my life.

∎

Emotional Triage

I have faith in myself and my abilities.
I am calm under pressure; I know what to do.

▪

I handle any issue that arises with confidence and grace.

▪

My mind is flexible and I am open to new experiences.
I am adaptable. I am open to change.

▪

I have been well trained and I have what I need
to do a good job for my patients.

▪

I am always learning. My practice is constantly improving.

▪

I stay in curiosity. I am not quick to judge.

▪

My mind is clear and my heart is peaceful today.

▪

I am undistracted. It is easy for me
to prioritize my patients' needs.

▪

I am grateful for the connections
I have with my patients and coworkers.

Affirmations

■

I listen keenly to my intuition.
My intuition sees what my eyes cannot.
I trust my inner voice.

■

I have amazing coworkers.
We communicate well and value the job we do together.
I am on a great team.

■

I do the best I can, and I release the outcome.

■

I handle all obstacles with grace and calm.

■

I can do this. This is tough, but so am I.

■

I do what I can when I can.

■

I am trained to do what most cannot. I joyfully do my part.

Emotional Triage

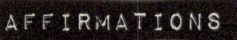

Post-Shift

My purpose here is not to fix it all.

▪

It is safe for me to lay down today's burdens.

▪

It is my turn to relax. I can release control.

▪

I have reported off to capable hands; now I can rest.

▪

I forgive myself for any shortcomings today.
They are a chance to learn and to do better next time.

▪

I am part of a Grand Plan. I proudly do my part.

▪

By consistently doing my best, I honor myself.
I also know that my best is not always enough
to change the situation. This is not a reflection of me,
but a product of a difficult situation
that is resistant to change. I persist by doing my best.

Affirmations

■

I do my best and I release my control over the outcome.

■

I have done enough for today. I can rest and let go.

■

I maintain my healthy boundaries.

■

I listen to my body's signals.

■

I give more when I have enough to give.

■

It is now time to turn my attention inwards. It is time to take care of me and those who are closest to me.

■

I reclaim my Energy. I call it back to me.

■

I fill my lungs with fresh air and slowly release my breath.
I exhale whatever feels heavy.

■

My turn to carry this weight has ended.
I release it and feel myself relax and rest.

Emotional Triage

■

I easily identify any Energies I may have collected today.
These are not mine! I shake them off,
and I feel my peacefulness grow.

■

I feel empowered, relaxed, and hopeful.

■

I am calm. My shoulders feel light.
My heart is peaceful. I feel joy.

■

I know myself. I trust myself.

■

I am well grounded.

■

I feel myself smile. I am safe. I am home within my mind.

CHAPTER 10

Visualizations

Visualizations, like affirmations, require some Energy input and faith from you. Whether you buy into the power of visualization or not, you are already doing them. Don't believe me? That mindless daydream you have when you allow your mind free rein—that's a visualization. When you are feeling anxious, playing out in your mind all the possible ways a situation could go, that's a visualization. The difference here is that you design, or follow, a visualization intended to help and promote your well-being. Imagine the possibilities for improving your life! All that is required is a little diligent conditioning of your thought patterns. You will get out what you put into your visualizations (what you think about, you bring about!). So give it a try. Once again, it is just you and yourself in your mind. So don't be afraid to go in there.

Create a detailed visualization of where you want to be or what you want to be doing. See yourself succeeding and feeling good. See yourself overcoming your obstacles. Infuse your Energy and your feelings into it. The more you do a particular visualization, the more real it will become. You will begin to feel it. Since your mind believes what you tell it repeatedly, it will provide you with some of the sensory experiences of your visualization. Allow yourself to be immersed completely. It's trippy, but it's true. The human mind is so powerful. For help with this, just do a YouTube search for "visualization meditation"—you will have no shortage of inspiration.

The following exercises are examples of visualizations to help you protect your Energy and emotions. They will give your mind a framework on which to hang some of the difficult stuff that you inevitably encounter. They are a backbone of sorts for the Energetic perspective that you must hold. Review them regularly so your mind knows the feel of them by memory. That way when you need them, they will be right there with you, wherever you are. You can make a micro-habit out of doing visualizations also. You do not need a lot of time to get all Zen. Just give yourself a couple of minutes to quiet your mind, take some big, controlled breaths, and allow yourself to focus solely on the visualization. You could literally do these in two minutes!

Visualizations

Cords and Conduits

Cord cutting is a very well-known visualization exercise. Its basic purpose is to disconnect or "cut" the emotional and Energetic power cords that bind you to another person or situation. It is for those poor souls whose Energy is so tangled into another's that they cannot call it back to them. There is no shame in being one of those poor souls. We all are there from time to time. When the Energetic connection to a person or event has become like a cord, sinewy and thick, it must be excised, lest the cord continue to draw from and steal your Energy. Often, the cord attaches to the chakra, or Energy center, that correlates with that emotion. (I won't go into detail on this. But if the idea of emotional Energy centers piques your interest, read Caroline Myss's book, *The Anatomy of the Spirit*).

The cord-cutting visualization below is ideal for releasing yourself from the patient scenarios that you can't seem to forget. The ones that haunt you. The ones whose circumstances were so bad that you leave them out when your family asks you about your day. You may be interested to know that studies have shown that the initial response to an emotion lasts only ninety seconds. Any additional time we have spent dwelling on them is us investing our Energy into sustaining that emotional response. Our continued Energetic investment keeps these emotions alive and stewing within us. We continue to be affected by them because we keep nurturing and sustaining them. A cord-cutting visualization can free you from this. It also works for ex-husbands, bad bosses, and any other situation or person you need to separate yourself from. Not that I would know (wink).

There are several guided meditations out there, on YouTube or even apps, that can talk you through a cord cutting. This one, like everything else in this book, is my version to get you started. Look around for one that works for you if this one doesn't resonate with you. A cord-cutting visualization is particularly impactful at the end of your day to help you release the drama from your shift. Or use this throughout the day to rid yourself of the bad juju of a particular patient or situation.

Cord-Cutting Visualization

Get yourself comfortable in a safe and quiet place. Sit cross-legged or sit in a chair with your feet on the floor and your arms supported so you don't have to think about them.

Visualizations

Above all, be comfortable so you can relax your body and mind. Now, close your eyes and focus on your breathing. In, then out. Try to take some cleansing breaths, but don't force it. It might take you a few minutes here to relax and open yourself enough to get a full breath in. Be patient with yourself; you are not in a hurry. Begin when you are ready.

Visualize yourself standing across from the person or situation that has a hold on you. Focus on your Energy. Where is it going? Where in your body is it leaving you? See the Energy leaving you as a golden thread, or cord, attaching to the person or situation across from you. See it actively pulsating away from you. This is your life force, and you are giving it away. You may notice if there is Energy flowing toward you as well. Is it a different color or texture than your own? This is the Energy from the other person, or situation, infiltrating into you. Using your higher mind for perspective and observe this scene. What do you see?

Go to the center of the cord between you and the person or situation you are bound to. Hold it in your hand and feel the vibration of the Energy pulsing through it. Pull a knife from your pocket and cut through that cord. Saw through it if you have to. It does not bleed and it does not hurt. It is just a clean cut. See the golden Energy moving from the cut end through the cord and back into you. This is the power returning to you that you have been giving away. Feel it replenishing you. See the other Energy returning to its owner, the cord drying and disappearing as it empties. The separation is complete, and you are whole again. Enjoy this for a few moments before you continue with your day.

Energetic Personal Protective Equipment (EPPE) Visualization

Do this visualization with me. The more you do it, the more your mind will fill in any details and gaps, and you will make it your own. I often do this visualization just before I get out of the car before my shift or as I am walking into my department. You will find the right time for you.

The weather report this morning says there is 100% chance of rain. As you look out your front door you see a downpour. In the entryway of your home is a coat rack with a yellow rain jacket hanging by its hood. It is a substantial jacket of excellent quality. You can see that it is fully lined; it will keep you warm and dry. Pick up the coat off the hook and put it on, one arm, then the other. It is your perfect size. It is long enough, down to your mid-thigh, and the cuffs on the sleeves hit just above your

Visualizations

knuckles. You adjust the fit so your shoulders are positioned comfortably and button the snaps down the front, then pull the hood up over your ears and hair. As you step out into the rain you can hear the raindrops pelting the hood of the jacket. They hit your shoulders like little bombs being dropped from the heavens. Wow, it's really coming down. You decide to stand in the rain for a moment, admiring the storm and its power.

You return to the safety of your covered doorway, water dripping off your coat. You carefully take your raincoat off to prevent yourself from getting wet. The outer shell is drenched, and the beads of rain fall to the ground from the edges of the coat. You shake the coat out and the particles of rain disperse away from you in a spray. They catch flight and disappear into the wind. You hang the coat back on its rightful hook. It will hang there loyally until you need it again. It's only now that you realize that you are completely dry. A quality raincoat, indeed.

Follow me on this analogy. When you wear a raincoat amid a downpour, you can feel the vibration of the raindrops hitting you through the outside of the coat. They don't hurt you, they just drop. But because you feel and hear the vibration, you are aware it is raining. You notice the drops of rain collecting in the folds of the outer layer of the coat. In this analogy and visualization, they are representations

Emotional Triage

of other people's pain and trauma. They are other people's problems and burdens. They are heavy droplets of other people's Energy. Sometimes the drops pool and begin to drip off the jacket as the rain keeps falling. But you are warm and dry; the rain has not soaked through to your skin. You are untouched. Your own Energy is safe and strong and unaffected.

Please notice also that in this analogy I did not put you in a suit of armor, or Kevlar, or even a plastic bubble. That is intentional. It is important for you to feel and to be aware of each drop as it hits you. This will keep you tuned in and feeling compassion for your patients. It will keep your connection to them strong and honest. This connection is able to fill up, or empty out, those all-important Energy tanks that we keep talking about.

Think of the raincoat analogy as your Energetic Personal Protective Equipment. Your EPPE. Just like our masks and face shields and gloves enable us to feel safe and to still give care, your EPPE allows you to connect without commingling your Energy. This is the emotional and Energetic separation that we should have with the people we interact with. We are aware of their struggles and we can feel the

Visualizations

vibration of their pain. But it does not soak into our skin and penetrate our core Energy.

When you are preparing to go to work, after your pre-shift affirmations, visualize putting on your raincoat. Visualize wearing it throughout your shift. Feel it against your skin. Pop up your hood before you walk through the doorway into a patient's room. Zip it up before having a difficult conversation with a family member or a co-worker. Be intentional about your visualization. Understand that you are putting on your EPPE to protect your Energy. Take it off and shake it out (literally) if it starts to feel too heavy and if the drops are beginning to soak through.

CHAPTER 11

Rituals

We are all drawn to rituals even without realizing. Leaving Christmas cookies out for Santa, a cigarette after sex, or even Happy Hour—these are all rituals. While the above-mentioned practices may be a bit clichéd, they are widely accepted rituals within our culture. The great thing about a ritual is that it can make even the simplest thing feel sacred. What is important about a ritual is not the practice itself but the emotion and the intention behind it.

As a ritual is performed again and again with intention, its importance becomes established. I challenge you to create a few rituals tailored just for you. In creating these rituals, you establish a sacred way to honor yourself. I will take you through how to create a ritual in just a minute. First let me tell you my practice so you can see what I mean.

I have a few rituals I have established to honor myself and engage in multilevel self-care. Feel free to steal them if any piece of them resonates with you.

Emotional Triage

I have a morning ritual. I get up early and start my day with a big glass of cool water. While the water is boiling for my French-pressed coffee, I stretch and do a couple basic strength exercises. When my coffee is done, I pour it into my favorite mug (a gift from a dear friend) in the shape of a flamingo. It's a little thing, but the flamingo brings me a little joy every morning. I sit down at our dining room table and light a candle. With the candle and the coffee, I enjoy a few sacred moments of quiet prayer and visualization. I review my affirmations, and sometimes I journal. Then I open my iPad, and I write. That is how I am writing this book, in fact. I have created a sacred time each morning, carved out just for me, my higher needs, and my goals. Even though I get up so early, I am energized the whole day because of this self-honoring ritual I have done. Even if the whole day goes to shit at work, I have already accomplished some of my personal daily goals, and I have made myself a priority. I have also achieved several levels of self-care with just my daily morning ritual!

I got the idea for my morning ritual from a book I read a while back called *The Miracle Morning*, by Hal Elrod. Elrod advises getting up a little early each morning and going through a routine similar to the one I describe above. How much time you allow depends on your personal needs.

Rituals

He says you can even do it in as little as six minutes a day. I highly recommend the read if you are inclined toward personal growth on any level. At first, the thought of getting up any earlier than I already did for my 5:30 a.m. shift sounded miserable. But now, I have grown to really enjoy it, and I look forward to my morning ritual. I love the feeling of my calm, quiet house. All my crazy kiddos are sleeping. The world is still. No one needs anything from me. It is a little piece of stolen time.

Another ritual I greatly enjoy on a regular basis is an evening candlelit bath. It's no surprise here that this is a great way to relax after work. But I want to stress that it is the intention behind the practice that makes it sacred. Thankfully both my husband and I recognize that an evening bath is an intentional, sacred ritual for me. It is understood that he is in charge of the kids during this time, and I am free to lock the door and quietly call my Energy back to me after a taxing day at work. Usually, I sit cross legged in the tub and stretch my hips and back. I often read or journal, or sometimes listen to a meditation track—whatever I feel like I need to do to come back to my center. I can release the day and refocus on my home and my family after expending my Energy at work. There is also some beautiful symbolism,

Emotional Triage

I suppose, to wash the day off my body, while I cleanse my mind and Energy as well.

I challenge you to create some rituals for yourself. Maybe you like to take a walk in the evenings. Maybe you take your dog out in the backyard and play frisbee. Maybe your ritual is to make a home-cooked meal. It could be anything that serves you (and possibly those you love) and is done with the intention of making it a sacred practice in your life. Identify it and create your intention. Be aware that you do your ritual to honor yourself. Acknowledging that you are doing it to honor yourself is self-affirming. It is something that is for you. Be mindful about it, and don't do it on autopilot. Make it feel luxurious, or even decadent, whatever it is. Bless your ritual and yourself as you perform it. Tweak it as needed to suit your multilevel self-care needs day to day.

CHAPTER 12

Quiet Headspace Time

Quiet self-reflection time is so important, given our overly stimulated lives. If you have kids, then I'm especially talking to you. My house is almost never quiet. Even in our work lives, the buzzes, beeps, and constant alarms of patient care equipment have infiltrated our quiet subconscious—not to mention our own internal alarms and reminders that go off related to our patients' needs. As a result of all this noise, it is imperative to have quiet time by yourself throughout the day wherever you can find it.

Most days, after a long shift, I sit in silence in my car for a few minutes before I turn the key in the ignition. (PSA: Please lock your car doors when you get safely inside.) When I climb in the car and close the door, the depth of silence and stillness envelopes me. The stark contrast of my surroundings hangs thick around me. I can hear and feel my own heartbeat. I am suddenly very aware of my breathing.

Emotional Triage

As I take a few minutes in the quiet for myself, I feel my shoulders drop down from their elevated and ever-ready position. My breath begins to slow and deepen. It even feels like my inner ear, which has been vibrating all day, softens and releases its tension. I am aware that my body responds immediately to my new surroundings. Only in moments like this, when my mind quiets and my body recovers, am I able to hear my inner self. I do a quick check-in with my Energy, my emotions, and my body. How am I? Usually, my answer back to myself is "I'm tired." Sometimes it's "I'm angry." Or "I'm sad." Or even "I'm feeling frustrated." Occasionally, I don't have an answer as to how I am. "I am numb." The important thing is the asking. The asking gives permission for my inner self to bring forth an honest, even vulnerable, answer. Read that sentence again. I give myself permission. This is so important. Permission to feel. Even as I am writing this, I am only now understanding that that is really what I am giving to myself.

Once I have identified these emotions and called them out for what they are, then I can begin to process them. If I don't take the time to see them, then they may begin to fester. Emotions will demand to be acknowledged, one way or another. They can morph into demons if they are left in the dark too long.

Quiet Headspace Time

Now let me be clear: I am not encouraging you to have a full-on pity party in your car. What I am encouraging is that you let down your guard in your safe and private corner (or car). Allow yourself to be vulnerable and to acknowledge, "Gosh, that was hard," or "Damn it, that was unfair." This is where you can unpack the raw emotion of your day and let it air out. Call it whatever it was. Only after you acknowledge it can you begin to process it in a positive way and move forward. This is what emotional self-care looks like.

Unless you are running late to pick up a kid from daycare or some other time-sensitive engagement, give yourself a few minutes in a quiet safe space to climb down out of that crazy tree you've been up in. Nobody will miss you for the five or so minutes it takes you to reconnect with yourself. This is a good time to review your post-shift affirmations. Visualize removing your EPPE and shake that shit out! If you find one person or situation is particularly affecting you, try a cord-cutting visualization and reclaim your Energy.

These few sacred moments alone will create a separation between your work life and your home life. Keep a clear delineation, and don't contaminate your home with work Energy (or germs from work—gross).

CHAPTER 13

Uncluttered Spaces

From the day I first binged Marie Kondo's show on Netflix, I felt a little "spark of joy" and hope within my heart. I really struggle keeping a tidy house. Honestly, I struggle to even keep a clean house, let alone tidy. On the bright side, I'm sure that the microbes at work in my home are building an amazing immune system within my children. I saw a Facebook meme recently about how cleaning a house with little kids at home is like brushing your teeth while eating Oreos. This meme totally summarizes my housekeeping experiences over the last several years.

I have always considered myself a lazy perfectionist. I love it when things are just so. I just usually don't spend the time and energy to make them that way. I casually studied *feng shui* many years ago. Its basic premise is to organize your home in such a way as to allow for harmonious Energetic flow throughout the space. I will not get overly woo woo here, but I did perceive the benefits for myself. Energy stagnates in an overly cluttered space. I have become very aware that I feel anxious and irritated when I'm surrounded by too much stuff, or too much out-of-place stuff. The old adage "cluttered home, cluttered mind" may come into play here.

Over the years I have even developed a habit of rearranging my furniture every few months in an unconscious attempt at clearing out the Energy in the room. I move the couch to the other side of the room and discover three dimes, two mismatched socks, fruit snack wrappers, a valentine from last year, and a warren of dust bunnies. Sure, the mere act of removing these things from under the couch is satisfying. Tell me cleaning that up isn't therapeutic. But I swear there is something about changing the layout or the design of a room that fills up my Energy tank a bit. It just feels fresh and new again. Open the windows and the doors and let the wind blow through the room. This may sound ridiculous, but it is strangely invigorating to me. Try it for yourself and see what you think.

Basket Case

My family and I have a knack for having too many things. I start out with the best of intentions. Everything starts out with a designated location, but after they are used, they almost never find their way back there. Using my micro-habit approach and honoring my practical self-care, I spend just a couple minutes in the morning and a couple minutes in the evening picking a few things up. Depending on the damage done to the home throughout the day, sometimes this is enough to take the edge off. Sometimes it is not.

In an attempt to have everything neatly in its place, I've even resorted to the basket/cubby system. You know, the one where you go buy a whole bunch of cute containers to stylishly hide all your shit in plain sight. The idea here, I guess, is to make it easier to put stuff away. This enables you to store your crap with effortless style—Pinterest-worthy, even. Honestly, this is the best system I have found. When things are put away, my house looks great. However, I should warn you that this system also makes it very easy for my four-year-old daughter to effortlessly dump and scatter the contents of said "stylish basket " onto the living room floor. No, I have not documented any of these catastrophes on social media, by the way (#RealLife). And the stuff never goes back into the basket the same way. I swear all of it fit in there before! Next, I resort to desperately stuffing it somewhere, anywhere. Just get it out of my sight. Occasionally, a "less is more" approach wins me over. A black garbage bag headed to the Goodwill is the only solution I can find in this situation to relieve myself of the anxiety surrounding the shit scattered at my feet. Pack it up and toss it. Enough is enough.

It can be so defeating, a perpetual cyclone of life that comes to undo all that you just spent your time and precious energy doing. I think the answer here might be just to have less stuff. But this is really difficult with small children. The stuffed animals and kid's meal toys alone could overwhelm a household. If you live alone, you will have more control over this. If you are a multi-tasking parent like me—drowning in crayons, pet rocks, and naked Barbies with tangled hair—just know that this period of clutter is temporary. Keep your perspective. Hang on and breathe through it. You are not alone.

CHAPTER 14

Avoiding Black Holes

Another way to take care of your ever-important Energetic environment is to avoid the Black Hole People. They will suck the Energy right out of you. You know who I'm talking about. These are the people who every day are looking for something to be upset about. They are looking desperately for a reason to have a bad day. They are poised for it. It's no surprise that they always seem to find what they are looking for. These people are toxic to your good Energy. If you are not paying attention, they will suck you right down into their negative spiral. Black Holes are the ultimate Energy leaks.

The first step is being able to identify them. This may or may not be easy for you, depending on your current level of awareness, although some are very easy to spot. When you are accustomed to feeling a more elevated level of Energy, you will begin to feel the difference when they are present. I may be presenting this in a way that is new to you.

Emotional Triage

You may know Black Holes by their various other names, like passive-aggressive, narcissist, martyr, or Eeyore, to name a few. A tell-tale sign of a Black Hole Person is when you start to feel like you can't ever do enough for them. They always need more, a literal Energy suck. You will never be enough for them. They are inherently difficult to please. Or, if they are pleased, they immediately demand more. They can't get enough of your Energy. Thus, I call them Black Hole People, bottomless pits never to be filled. Be kind to them but stop trying to please them. Do not spend your Energy here.

Often Black Holes are very good and well-meaning people. They may be very friendly, even helpful. They are probably trudging through their own days, dealing with a very real, acute level of burnout or an Energy deficit. Maybe they are sick or in pain and can't manage their own Energy leaks. They could just be stuck in a very negative cycle. Maybe they don't even know what it is like to not be an Energy suck, they have been at it for so long. Maybe they are just an asshole. There are all kinds of reasons people become Black Holes and subsequently feel the need to fill themselves with the Energy of others. These things are perpetuated in families and social groups too. You get used

Avoiding Black Holes

to and become what is around you. "Misery loves company," remember? But also remember that they probably don't even know what they are doing. They are generally unaware of the Energetic world and their place in it. So again, be kind, but don't stay long. There is nothing for you there but exhaustion and disappointment.

Most of us don't get to pick our coworkers or our patients, so inevitably there will be a few Black Holes for you to maneuver around on a daily basis. Recognize them for what they are. Avoid them if you can. Don't give them your power. If you struggle with this, try doing the Energetic Personal Protective Equipment visualization exercise, or even the cord-cutting visualization we talked about earlier. These are scenarios where your EPPE may come in handy, so protect yourself.

CHAPTER 15

Prioritize Sleep

I never had a nap I didn't like. I recognize that telling you to get a good night's sleep is not earth-shattering news for you. You are an educated person, and you are likely encouraging your patients to rest and sleep regularly. It is how our bodies build, repair, and heal. It fills up your physical energy tank. Duh, I know.

What your highly analytical mind may not know is that science is finding convincing evidence of a connection with sleep and the brain's processing of recent emotional experiences. This is known as "sleep-dependent emotional brain processing." According to a 2009 UC Berkeley study, the lack of sleep may have an impact on your mood and mental health. More recent studies are confirming these findings, noting that "lack of sleep significantly influences emotional reactivity." Any parent of a toddler who has not napped can confirm these findings. But it is nice to know that our beloved scientists and researchers are tracking it, with brain scans and all.

Emotional Triage

The takeaway is to recognize that when you are tired, you are more likely to feel overwhelmed and on your way to burnout. When you feel like the world is crashing down around you, you hate your job, your life is terrible—stop and get perspective here. Check in with yourself. No, your life doesn't suck; you've just had a long day and you're tired. Try not to take yourself or your circumstance(s) too seriously when you are low on sleep. Like I tell my little girls, and often have to remind myself, "a grumpy girl is a sleepy girl."

Be aware of your sleep deficit and plan to go to bed early. Napping can be good too. You've got to catch up somewhere. I love a long nap on my days off. I wake up feeling renewed, and there's definitely some emotional brain processing going on there! It is very difficult to get an accurate perspective on anything when you are tired. When it seems like the world is stacked against you, sometimes you just need to crawl in bed, pull the covers up under your chin, and let yourself doze off. Sweet dreams, darling!

CHAPTER 16

Be Silly

Our work environment can be intense. It is easy to get overwhelmed with stress, even within a short period of time. We must be ready for anything. One minute we're quietly catching up on some charting, and the next we're working a "code blue" down the hall. Ever ready and in constant anticipation, is it any wonder we develop a dark sense of humor? It is basically a survival skill for the medical field. There is an emotional need to find a release to the tension. We can't be wound so tight all the time. A little levity is needed to diffuse the situation. That's where silliness comes in.

Children are great at being silly. Just watch them play together for a few minutes and they find ways to be creative and provide entertainment for each other. They are not afraid to look silly in front of their friends or to be the reason people are laughing. Indeed, that is the point. But as we grow up, we begin to take ourselves so seriously. The jobs we do are serious. We hold lives in our hands. But too often we lose our natural inclination to find the little joys and giggles hiding in our daily tasks. These are missed opportunities for connection with our coworkers (social self-care, anyone?). These little silly moments are humanizing and help us to let down our guard. They can endear people to each other, even if there are a few eye rolls. Here are a few examples of what I mean.

I work with an anesthesiologist who likes to tell really bad corny jokes as he is putting his patients to sleep on the operating table. Since I have worked with him often, I have heard most of these jokes and usually roll my eyes at him. But the patient in our care has never heard them. No matter how bad the joke, the patient drifts off to sleep under anesthesia with a giggle and a lighthearted notion in their mind. This is otherwise a very stressful time for a patient. This doctor uses humor to diffuse his patient's fear.

Last year I took a trip to the zoo with my family. My kids love our hometown zoo, and we go fairly often. I was taking pictures of the kiddos looking at the animals and documenting the experience so we could look back on the day and remember what a good time we had together. Later that evening I was glancing through the photos I had taken.

Be Silly

Sure, there were a few of the kids. There was one of them in the red panda exhibit and another standing next to the meerkats. But, to my surprise, most of the pictures I had taken were of the flamingos. Whoops, mom fail. Without even thinking about it, I had become mesmerized by the flamboyant birds and had taken more pictures of them than I had of my children. It never even occurred to me that I liked flamingos all that much. But they are kind of ridiculous, I love their color, and, huh, they just make me happy!

That is when it all started, I think. I hesitate to call it an obsession, although others have described it that way. I bought myself a scrub cap with pink flamingos all over it. (Side note: Scrub caps to the OR nurse are a sacred thing. We love them. They are a required piece of uniform suitable for the sterile and sub-sterile areas. But they are the only real piece of flair we get. Everything else is hospital issued and just like everyone else's.) Anyway, the well-made cap had a white background with big pink flamingos, and it was finished off with a black satin bow. I wore it to work that Friday. I got lots of compliments. It was a little over the top, but it was so fun. I smiled a lot that day. I decided that I would wear that flamingo scrub cap every Friday (or at least my work Friday, which is sometimes Thursday) to celebrate the end of a busy week. And so, Flamingo Friday was born. Ever since that first Flamingo Friday, all sorts of fabulous flamingo-y things have been happening. Several of my coworkers decided that they liked the idea, so they came to work in flamingo scrub caps too!

Flamingos are appearing all over the surgical department. Text messages are sent to me with flamingo emojis, and little notes appear on my desk with hand-sketched flamingos from my nurses. One of my favorite surgeons told me jokingly the other day, when his case was delayed, "Put your flamingo hat on, and go take care of it!" Apparently, my flamingos and I have a reputation for getting things done. I am now the crazy flamingo lady, and Flamingo Friday is in full effect. Yes, it is ridiculous and that, my friends, is exactly the point.

Fun fact: A group of flamingos is called a *flamboyance*. This makes me love them even more.

CHAPTER 17

Hydration

As healthcare professionals, we are used to thinking about hydration in terms of electrolyte imbalances and skin turgor. We scan the patient's lab results and double check orders for maintenance fluids. It's all very clinical. We note that our patient's urine output has significantly decreased from yesterday and dive into the chart to check labs for kidney function results. Maybe the aid forgot to record an output from this morning? These output numbers just couldn't be right.

Conversely, what do you figure is your urine output is for a shift? I know many of us go most of a shift without peeing. If one of our patients did that, we would be concerned, on the phone asking for an order for a straight catheter. Don't get the bladder scanner out just yet! There is a more obvious reason for your lack of urine.

You are dehydrated!

Emotional Triage

If you are like me, and I know you are, you run on a steady supply of coffee to keep you going. Then, after you get home for the night, maybe you have a drink or two to help you unwind. A jammy red wine for me please! Seriously, there are some days I know I have had no water! Straight from coffee all day to wine at home for a dinner party all evening. Sigh. Okay, so maybe you drink iced tea or soda. It's not really much better. My point is none of this is water. It is literally a nutrient in itself. The beverages listed above are all diuretics. I recognize (thank you, renal experts) that something is better than nothing. But let's agree that these are probably not the ideal choices for optimal hydration.

Studies are finding a significant link between our bodies' hydration, our cognitive function, and especially (here's the kicker) our mood. Even our short-term memory is affected by dehydration. And I'm not talking about severe dehydration here. Even a small amount of dehydration (1–2%) is proven to have negative effects on our emotional state and long-term health, like increased incidences of chronic hypertension and stroke. This is according to the *British Journal of Nutrition*, January 2013, with other articles in agreement.

Hydration

So here's the simple micro-habit I have made for myself to prevent all the negative effects of dehydration. I do it every day, and now it is part of my routine. A micro-ritual, even.

I wake up and head to the kitchen, and I drink a very tall glass of water. Usually, it is out of my favorite 1-liter water bottle that I have strategically left on the counter from the night before. I fill it up, at least halfway, and guzzle. Sometimes I fill up a mason jar. I vary it sometimes and squeeze some lemons in if I have them available. Delicious. If I'm in the mood, I will warm it up. But mostly, it's just about getting a large amount of water down my gullet every single day before I do anything else. How much water? I'm not exactly measuring it out. As much as I can comfortably consume without feeling like I'm waterboarding myself, but at least 500 ml. Then I fill my water bottle up to the top and put it in my go-bag to sip on throughout my shift. My strategy is this: Even if I only drink that initial 500ish ml, and 1 L over the next twelve hours, I can likely find another 500 ml somewhere to make it to my goal. But, hey, even 1.5 L isn't that bad. It all starts with that first dose of hydration therapy first thing in the morning (or whenever you wake up, night shifters).

Emotional Triage

A few minutes after I drink all that water, I feel less groggy, even without coffee, which of course comes very shortly after the water. I notice my digestive system waking up. I feel like I've done a small thing to prioritize myself, giving my body something that it needs (physical self-care). It is a small victory, I know. Let's celebrate the small victories. They are worth it.

CHAPTER 18

Personal Anthems

You must have a personal anthem! You know, a fight song dedicated to you and your fabulousness. Your very own rallying cry. Maybe you have one already, and you're nodding your head because you know exactly what I'm talking about. Awesome, good for you! If you don't have one, do these visualizations with me, and let's find you one!

You're standing in front of the mirror, wearing your favorite outfit. Looking fierce! You assume the power stance. Hands on your hips, feet shoulder width apart. You are strong and confident. You look deep into your eyes in the mirror. Look at that determination! You give yourself a little nod and a wink. You definitely say, "Bring it!" This is what your personal anthem should make you feel like every time you hear it.

Here's another one to try. See yourself poised to take the field in your team's home stadium. You can hear the crowd in the stands. They are cheering and stomping their feet in anticipation. The sound reaches a fevered pitch. Your personal anthem starts to play. This is your cue to step into their view. You confidently stride out onto the field. Slowly now, give the people a good show. They are thrilled to see you. Your anthem and their cheers fill your ears.

The above scenarios are how your personal anthem should make you feel—emboldened and full of potential! It's a pep talk for yourself set to music. All you've got to do is push play, and you've got a little something extra to get you over the hump.

My personal anthem is "SuperWoman" by Alicia Keys (thank you, Alicia!). I put that song on and a cape magically appears on my shoulders. And yes, it does blow gently in the wind. I take my power stance and I see that "S on my chest, Oh yes." I am a Superwoman. I just needed a little reminder.

Feel free to use my song as your anthem if it speaks to you. You can find it, and all of my girl Alicia's other songs on Apple Music, YouTube, and I'm sure everywhere else. She came out with another song recently that is dedicated to healthcare heroes (wait, that's us!). It's called "Good Job."

Personal Anthems

I can't hear it without feeling proud of all the work that we do. Anyway, I digress; find yourself a song!

Here is a list of a few that might hit you (they date me if nothing else):

- "I Will Survive"—Gloria Gaynor
- "Roar"—Katy Perry
- "Lose Yourself"—Eminem
- "Get Up Stand Up"—Bob Marley
- "We Are the Champions"—Queen

CHAPTER 19

Dance It Out, Sing It Out

I have found that music is one of those subtle things that can influence our work environment in a big way. I often start the shift during our team's morning huddle with something bouncy and motivating over the speaker. While they are setting up their operating rooms and before patients are anywhere near, my teams are singing along and tapping their toes to the same beat. It is a simple way to unify ourselves, to begin our day headed together in the right direction. On the days where I get busy and forget to put some music on, somebody will mention, "It's too quiet out here" or "Put on something to change up the energy." It's like the music can carry us a bit and make the work feel a little easier.

I have music in my head all the time. I find myself singing or humming a random song (sometimes my anthem) as I do mindless things. Sometimes I throw a little booty shake down too. Hey, I'm not proud. There's nothing wrong with a little ad-libbed dance routine at the nurses' station. It feels good to shake out the tension that permeates around me.

One time, I walked past a scrub sink where a surgeon was scrubbing his hands before surgery. I was singing along to something, he nodded appreciatively and sang a few lines with me. Another doctor I know plays a killer playlist over the operating room's Bluetooth speaker while he operates, so his whole surgical team can hear it. His operating rooms are typically a low-stress environment. His surgical teams work efficiently and happily, and his cases go smoothly too. Win-win!

Music (and dance) can lift us up, or even help us process our thoughts and emotions. Again, it is just a little thing, but it can make a big difference. Incorporating a little music can diffuse tension and help with mental focus and stamina. When a song pops into my mind, I feel like it's my brain's way of taking a mini break, while my body handles whatever mundane task it must before my brain gives my body its next instruction. Music helps everything flow better.

Admittedly, you may not be able to work in a department that allows a little bit of music like mine. Maybe you could

Dance It Out, Sing It Out

put on some tunes in your break room, or put some music on for yourself through some earphones while you are on a break. You may find yourself singing (or whistling) a happy tune for the rest of the shift.

CHAPTER 20

Get a Life

There is so much more to you than this job you do. You are not your job or even your job title. Sure, sometimes we can enjoy those labels. We have worked hard for them, and we use them with pride. "I am a nurse." "I am a doctor." "I am . . . blah, blah, blah." But what else are you? We can sometimes exploit or neglect parts of ourselves by hiding behind these big labels.

Think of your life like a wagon wheel. Each spoke in the wheel represents a different facet of you. It's all those facets that make you sparkle! You are not a one-sided person, and you may have overdeveloped one or more areas of your life in your career pursuits. You have many strengths and gifts, and none of those strengths should overshadow the others. Just like the wagon wheel, each spoke (or strength) should be the same length so that it can carry the same load. This makes the wheel strong and balanced and allows the wheel to roll. The wheel can't roll efficiently if the spokes are different lengths. Not only is it an uncomfortable ride, but it is also more prone to breaking because of the imbalance. You are more prone to break if you are unbalanced too. If one aspect of your life has been overdeveloped, then other aspects will be weaker and the "wheel of your life" will not hold up under the weight of your stressors.

"Ah, yes," you say to yourself. "The old balanced life bit. I've heard this before." Yes, but are you actively working toward it? It can be easy to get lost in the daily routine and stuck in the demands of the work. Always pushing for more. But it is a routine that will wear you down, man! Your body and your mind need a rest from it. It's like that old proverb, "All work and no play makes Jack a dull boy." A dull boy probably bored out of his mind.

Let's break this down into a few basic categories of ways to bust you out of the work glut and start working toward that round, balanced wagon wheel kind of life.

Personal Growth

The mere fact that you have purchased this book and are reading it (thank you) tells me that you have some interest in personal growth. Personal growth has so many forms because, well, it's personal. There are so many ways to grow, but the simple fact is that *you must feed your brain.* Maybe you've considered going back to school or learning a new skill? Is there a short course or clinic you have been thinking about? Maybe you need to pay more attention to your spiritual development, or you need to focus on bettering your relationships. The areas for personal growth are endless. Just keep your eyes open for something that gives you a little spark or pulls on your heart. Pay attention when you feel it. It is trying to tell you something.

In general, reading books is a really good place to start or continue your personal growth. So, yay, you've already started. Books can broaden your perspective and generate new ideas. Once you've read a book it becomes part of you, and maybe it changes you in some way. And there is a book on just about every topic you can dream up. One of my favorite questions to ask friends is, "What are you reading?" It's just a simple little question with so many possibilities. But by asking this question, I'm really asking, "How are you growing? What are you feeding your mind? Who are you becoming?"

Sharing a reading list can be strangely intimate. Just sharing the titles you are reading allows insight into your inner thoughts and your inner world. (Pssst, I share my favorite reads at the end of the book.)

Books are great, too, because they are inexpensive, portable, and available in multiple formats. You can make a micro-habit out of them and take them in a little at a time. Or you can binge-read them. I consume most of my books via Audible on my commute to work. It kind of feels like cheating to not be reading, but hey, the information is getting into my brain, so . . . same-same.

Whether it is a course or a class or a book, I challenge you to dive into something to expand yourself. Only you will know what rabbit hole to fall into! As you learn, you will inadvertently push out the boundaries of your personal context and perspective. You may find that your Energy is expanding too. You may have a deeper well from which to draw your emotional endurance. Inevitably, the more you grow and learn, the more you will want to grow and learn. Keep going. It is a journey that never ends.

Hobbies & Creativity

I think of hobbies and creativity like chewing gum for your brain. It gives you a little something to do without

Get a Life

being all-consuming, and it keeps you from overthinking. Can you walk and chew gum? Good; you can pick up a hobby. Find something, anything, that brings you some joy, something completely outside of the healthcare scene. Get creative. Maybe your thing is fly-fishing; maybe it's spending time with foster kids. Maybe you have a passion for backpacking or have it on your bucket list to run a marathon. Find something that fills you up, and take a day off here and there for this new activity. Obviously, some hobbies are more consuming than others, so choose according to your interest and your current levels of energy. Don't overwhelm yourself. Work into it slowly if you must. You already have a lot going on. Simpler hobbies may include taking a quilting class, joining a book club, or taking a stand-up paddle board out for a spin. It's okay to be a little noncommittal for a while. The point is to find your thing, then treat yourself by going and doing it regularly.

Many hobbies engage your creativity too. If you find a hobby that gets your creative juices flowing, bonus points for you. Creativity feels like recess to me. Let your mind run out on the playground and have some fun. There are usually only a few rules in any creative endeavor and the rest you make up as you go along.

During the first several months of COVID, I taught myself embroidery. It was a great quarantine activity. Embroidery was something I had been aware of; my grandmother and her sisters were well versed in needle crafts. But I had never taken the time to learn it. I downloaded a how-to book (you can find anything online), learned a few stitches, and I was off to the races! I found it to be incredibly meditative. I could transcend the uncertainty of the world around me and just focus on pulling the colored thread through the fabric. Then I would plunge my needle back in again. I found myself getting lost in it in a good way. I was creating something beautiful out of a scrap piece of fabric and some thread. It was very satisfying and it kept me from overthinking during such a difficult time. Now, I have beautiful and memorable art pieces to show for my efforts from that strange time.

Adventures

Have you ever considered that planning a vacation can be almost as much fun as taking one? When we plan, we visualize ourselves doing that thing. As we've discussed before, your brain believes whatever you tell it. Visualizing yourself doing the things you will do on your vacation activates the same pathways in the brain that relate to actually doing those things. This is awesome because you get the positive effects of the visualization and get to enjoy doing them on your trip too! Plus, the anticipation can be so delicious. I love daydreaming about my next trip; it's like a mini-vacation.

I am in no way suggesting you only plan vacations. On the contrary, take them. Take many of them. They don't need to be fancy or even long. Just something new and stimulating to break you out of your everyday grind. Even a well-timed day off midweek to explore that little town you've never been to that is only an hour away can be amazing for your well-being. Day trips are a great escape.

I work with a group of young ICU nurses who are always taking off somewhere or getting back from some grand adventure. They post pictures all over their social media of their exploits. It's like looking at something out of *Travel + Leisure Magazine*. Backpacking in Big Sur, skiing in Tahoe, a road trip of the Southwest—all amazingly beautiful adventures and experiences. Sure, they are young and single, and likely without house payments, but they are out seeking adventure in their lives. I think they may be onto something here. They are actively and deliberately making time for their adventures and their friendships. Seriously, use your vacation days. What the hell have you been saving them for?

Think carefully about where you want to go and what you want to do. This sounds obvious, I realize. But don't pick the clichéd version of what you think a relaxing getaway should be. Don't go to Cabo and drown yourself in margaritas if that is not what your heart truly wants. Sure, relaxing poolside always sounds great for a few days. But after that, you've essentially beached yourself. Your mind and heart are not engaged. You're stuck in autopilot! Maybe all of this is what you need, but maybe it's not. Are you craving something more adventurous?

Some of my most memorable and rejuvenating getaways have been trips that have engaged my mind and my body. I have found over the years that often, and to my surprise, I crave something more adventurous. My monkey mind gets bored doing nothing for too long. Without even knowing it, I am searching for a new experience, a challenge. I credit my husband for being our family's ultimate trip planner.

I love to finish a vacation and feel a sense of accomplishment, and he knows it. It felt good to put on a pack and hike those twenty-five miles in the quiet of the California wilderness. It was a very connected cultural experience to adventure through the streets of Barcelona, living like a local for eight days. Every music festival and outdoor concert I can escape to is a time of transcendence. The music fills me, and I can ride the good vibes with hundreds of others. More recently, I skied for the first time in twenty-five years (and I didn't break a hip)! I remember smiling ear to ear, stretching my arms out wide and turning my face to the sun, as I glided down the mountain. I exhaled more completely on that mountain than I had in months.

Moments like these remind me of how much life we have to live. These moments spent just outside of my comfort zone make me grateful beyond measure. They make my heart overflow. My Energy tank is full. I usually come home physically tired, needing a day or two to recover before I go back to work. Sometimes I get the rest before I go back to work, sometimes I don't. But the adventure is always worth it.

Work hard, play hard. Repeat.

CHAPTER 21

Renewing Your Purpose

I find a fleeting moment of renewal as a nurse when I help a patient go to sleep under anesthesia. I hold the plastic oxygen mask against their mouth and cheeks. The milky propofol flows into their veins, and they look up at me. They look at me! I am the last piece of life as they know it before they drift into the great unknown of the anesthetic fog. Most are scared, even the tough ones. They glance into my eyes for reassurance, and then they close theirs. It is such a common moment in the life of an OR nurse. It is done many, many times in a day without incident or emergency. Yet it is always profound to me. I pray it will always have such an impact upon me. There is a very uncommon level of intimacy and trust that is shared in a fleeting moment like that when someone is so vulnerable. It's a beautiful and unguarded exchange with someone I barely know.

Moments like this are part of what drew me into nursing. They reconnect me to why I became a nurse in the first place.

Emotional Triage

I want to be a safe harbor for someone in a storm. I want to advocate for them, and I want to connect with them. I want to leave them better than I found them. If I am truly honest with myself, these are the root reasons of why I became a nurse.

Have you found your purpose? Why did you begin your journey into caring for others? I bet it wasn't for the money. In what small moments in the swirling chaos of your workday do you find a glimmer of your purpose? Have you lost track of it? Or maybe you need to redefine your purpose because it doesn't resonate with you any longer.

Take some time to reflect and journal on what your purpose is and identify ways to engage with your purpose more often.

CHAPTER 22

So Now You Know

If you've read this far, you now know more intimate details of my daily life and inner mind than most of my dear friends. As you can imagine, writing this book has been a deeply personal journey. Sometimes this book has been a journal, allowing me to reflect, and sometimes it's been a personal survival guide. Either way, I hope reading it has given you a piece of what you are searching for. This has been my journey, now it is time for you to take or continue with your own.

My journey as a woman and as a nurse is a work in progress, just like you. I will continue to do the things we have discussed. I will still get up a little early most mornings, chug some water, and begin my morning ritual. Have you made one yet? I will still be looking for ways to incorporate micro-habits and multilevel self-care into my day to keep me incrementally moving forward, in every direction, so that my life may be as balanced as possible. But I know my house will still be a mess, and I'm working on letting that go too. I will visit and revisit my affirmations, and I will write more as it suits me. So should you. I will pop up the hood on my EPPE before I go in to handle anything that might drain my Energy. I will identify what Energy is mine and what Energy is not, and I will release it so I will not be consumed by it. I will take quiet time to unpack my emotions. I will continue to be silly, and dance and sing and celebrate Flamingo Fridays. I will not take myself too seriously. I will continue to grow, evolve, create and adventure. And I hope that you will too, my friend.

Below are a few guidelines for going forward on your journey.

Guidelines for Going Forward

1. You are responsible for your physical energy. You are also responsible for your Energy, the Energy that is YOU. This means that you do what is necessary to protect and refuel your Energies. Advocate for them as if your life depends on it, because it does. Your physical and emotional health, as well as the quality of your life, depends on the refueling and protection of your Energies at all costs. Think of your Energies like a currency; spend them wisely.

So Now You Know

2. Now that you know about how your Energy affects others, you are obligated to be aware of what you are sending out to others. You have the ability to effect change, good or bad. You are now part of a secret society of good Energy propagators. Once you know, you know. So, act accordingly and be responsible for the Energy you project to the world. Share your light and your kindness. Give genuine compliments generously. Smile and laugh with others. Help when and where you can.

3. Use your intentions to honor yourself and to honor others. Small intentional gestures focused inwardly or outwardly can mean big changes. Do small things with big intentions.

4. Don't take yourself so damn seriously. You are here on purpose, yes, but you are also here for fun. Be silly. Enjoy your journey and allow your mind to play. You do not need to handle it all. Do your part diligently. Then let go.

5. Keep growing and caring for yourself on multiple levels. Keep evolving yourself. Like a fine wine, you should be getting better every year. Remember the wagon wheel and grow in a balanced way.

Emotional Triage

6. Get comfortable sitting with yourself in the quiet. Be yourself with yourself, and don't make judgments about who and what you should be. Just be. Then affirm your intentions as if you have already accomplished them. Visualize yourself doing the things you need to do in order to become the person you want to be.

If you come up with another guideline for going forward, send it to me! These are by no means exhaustive. Since we are in the digitally connected age, I can update future versions of this book for others to continue to enjoy their evolution. Like the guidelines, the rituals and techniques are endless and ever expanding too. So if you have found one that I didn't cover here and would like to enlighten me, please share!

On that note, I have so enjoyed the experience of writing and publishing this book. I am nearly certain this will not be my last attempt at this beautiful exchange with you. So, if there is an experience, an insight, or an idea you would like to share with me to add to a future work, I would love to hear from you.

Connect with the Author

Subscribe to my mailing list to connect, and get updates from me in your inbox at www.OliviaLovejoy.com.

Like and follow "Olivia Lovejoy, Author" on Facebook.

Follow on Instagram:
@olivia_lovejoy_rn_author.

Send an email to
OliviaLovejoywrites@gmail.com
to land in my inbox.

RESOURCES

My Reading List—A Very Informal Bibliography

As I have mentioned previously, what you read becomes a part of you. It opens your mind and changes the way you see the world. Here is a bibliography of sorts.

Some of what I have included in this book are just things I've learned along the way. I'm not sure of their source exactly. They have just become part of me. Others are certainly right off the pages of the titles I have listed. I've attempted to include proper references to the studies I have mentioned throughout. I greatly apologize for any inadequate citation, as I have erred on the side of having a more readable and impactful text than an overly documented scientific study.

My hope is that if you are intrigued by one concept or another that I have brought up, you can easily start your search on that topic precisely where my search began.

This list is a road map of sorts, for where I have journeyed so that you may walk along the same path should you choose. Only you will know where your search will take you, so enjoy the journey and keep growing.

We are only as good as the thoughts, ideas, and Energy that we allow into ourselves. I am grateful to these authors for sharing themselves with me, as I am grateful to you for allowing me to share with you.

The Anatomy of the Spirit by Caroline Myss

This book was written many years ago and it was the first to get me thinking about what Energy is, and how it shapes us and our experience in the world. Myss has written several other books as well on this topic, but I think this one is the place to start.

The Power of Intention by Wayne Dyer

This was one of the first books on this list that I read, some fifteen or more years ago. I credit Dyer for reinforcing Mom's sentiments of "what you think about you bring about" and helping me to evaluate how my thoughts and intentions could shape my life.

Resources

Eat Pray Love by Elizabeth Gilbert

Not exactly a self-help book, but Gilbert's memoir had a profound impact on me. Her emotional vulnerability, her search for the higher power within her, and her commitment to her own growth made me want to start searching too. The movie that came out a few years later is a watered-down version of what was an enriching journey experienced by the author. Read the book.

101 Power Thoughts by Louise Hay

This is an audio track of an hour's worth of great affirmations. It is a bit dated, but it remains my go-to when I feel like I need a little pick-me-up on my way into work. It gets me focused on gratitude and possibility.

Micro Habits by Brian Leger and *Atomic Habits* by James Clear

Two great books that introduced me to the power of moving forward in small increments. Leger's book is short and to the point, and this is where I found the five squats a day example. Clear's book is a more of a complete study of the power of small things over time. Both are great reads.

The Miracle Morning by Hal Elrod

Reading *The Miracle Morning* got me serious about carving out regular time for myself and my personal growth. In these little sections of stolen time, I have created some valuable routines and rituals for myself, and I also got my thoughts, emotions, and experiences organized into the words you are reading now.

The Worthy Project by Meadow DeVor

This book got me thinking about the subtle ways we choose to give away our Energy and disempower ourselves as well as about how real and regular self-care empowers us and affirms our self-worth. It was a great read.

The Source by Tara Swart MD, PhD

Dr. Swart's book is a crossroads of psychiatry, behavioral science, neuroscience, and spirituality. As a senior lecturer at MIT, she explores the science behind the power of your mind and the importance of your intention. I listened to it twice, then I had to buy the paperback and read it again.

You Must Write a Book **by Honoree Corder**

As you may have derived from the title, *Emotional Triage* would not have happened had I not read Honoree's book. I am grateful for her encouraging and instructional words, and for implanting the idea within me that one of you may benefit from hearing my story.

Other Notable Sources and Resources

National Suicide Prevention Lifeline
(800)-273-8255 (TALK), or text HELLO to 741741
CompassionFatigue.org by Patricia Smith

Patricia Smith's great website is packed with resources for those who are interested in compassion fatigue and how to work through it. She has been one of the key players leading the charge in advocating for those of us in caregiving professions. Her great TED Talk is embedded into the homepage. I recommend taking a look at her clear and informative presentation on compassion fatigue.

Loss, Grief, and Bereavement **by Barbara Rubel,
4th Edition (Elite Healthcare 2018).**

Also see GriefWorkCenter.com by Barbara Rubel

I encountered Barbara Rubel's work while working through a 32-hour CE requirement. The course was well thought out and covered the grief process across multiple cultures and age groups. It focused on how to support patients and families with loss and culminated in how to cope as caregivers when faced with repeated loss. This was where I first heard the term *compassion fatigue*. Rubel has included multiple self-assessments for determining if you or a friend may be experiencing compassion fatigue.

"Nursing on Empty: Compassion Fatigue Signs, Symptoms, and System Interventions" by Harris, Griffin, and Quinn (Lippincott Nursing Center 2017)

A very well written and frequently cited article that does a great job of defining burnout and compassion fatigue with examples of each. Also, they address root causes of these issues, like a nurse's loss of purpose and lack of spiritual connection. Suggestions are made for hospital leadership to educate and support staff to increase staff retention and emotional welfare.

"Mild Dehydration Impairs Cognitive Performance and Mood of Men" by Matthew Giano et al. (*British Journal of Nutrition* 2011)

The above study is important because it studied the effects of mild dehydration (which occur at only 1–2%) and its effects on cognitive function and mood.

CONCLUSION

This is the end, my friend. It is my deepest hope that you have enjoyed this book and that it has provided you with some inspiration and lift to keep you going, tomorrow and beyond. Writing it and sharing it with you has been my great privilege. If you are inclined to leave a review or tell a friend about this book, please do so with my appreciation.

Reviews on Amazon and other platforms are the lifeblood of independent authors. Leave a review so that others can find this work in their search results.

Yours,

Olivia Lovejoy, RN